THE
DESK JOB
SURVIVAL GUIDE

THE
DESK JOB
SURVIVAL GUIDE

EXERCISE AND NUTRITION
FOR THOSE WHO SIT ALL DAY

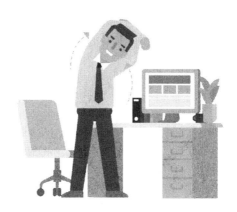

JAKE DERMER

For information about this title or to order other books and/or electronic media, contact the publisher:

Jake Dermer
www.doitatyourdesk.com
jderme2@gmail.com

Library of Congress Preassigned Control Number: In Process

ISBNs:
Print: 978-1-7331355-0-4
eBook: 978-1-7331355-1-1

Printed in the United States of America

Cover and Interior design: 1106 Design
Illustrations: Cristina Anichini

CONTENTS

PREFACE

DO YOU SPEND ALL DAY AT A DESK?

Does your job make staying fit difficult?

Sitting at a desk all day is hard. It takes a serious toll on your body and your mind. It is no exaggeration to say that sitting at a desk can make you overweight, depressed, and even physically debilitated. Luckily, if you are stuck at a desk all day and want to get healthy, you just picked up the right book.

Now, I'm not promising you a six-pack by the end of the week, but what I can offer is a realistic way to improve your overall quality of life by making you strong, lean, and pain free.

What most people don't realize about diet and exercise is that consistency is far more important than intensity. Over the course of a decade working in the fitness industry and studying health, I've developed this no B.S. resource that will help you develop a diet and exercise program that is practical and customized to you. And more importantly, it will fit easily into your busy corporate lifestyle.

Getting healthy takes work, but that doesn't mean it cannot be done conveniently.

CHAPTER 1

Don't buy into the B.S.

AS YOU ARE PROBABLY ALREADY AWARE, there is no magic pill—no revolutionary diet that will make you smarter and your skin always tan. There is no one trick to getting a six-pack and massive biceps—no effortless life hack for fixing your posture issues. Health and fitness take work, and the reason these things take work is because of our environment. Our environment shapes our minds and bodies to function in certain ways; you adapt to what you continually do. If you are a Sherpa living at high altitudes in the Himalayas, you become less susceptible to hypoxia when climbing Everest. If you are working a desk job that requires you to park it in front of a monitor for eight hours, you become less capable of maintaining good posture. We live in a soft environment, where our conflicts can be resolved by HR and inactivity is causing us more damage than activity.

Let's be honest: you have it easy—really easy.

If you are reading this, you probably aren't guessing where your next meal is coming from or if you'll be sheltered from the elements this evening. You are more likely at risk of seasonal affective disorder and chronic lower-back pain right now than you are of any immediate threat to your life. And the reason is clear: the modern environment we've created for ourselves.

Imagine you broke both your legs. If you work at a computer, there is a good chance you could work remotely until you healed. If you got hungry, you could order from literally any restaurant you could think of. Need to clean your house? Paint a room? Cut your hair? Clip a toenail? There's an app for that.

Nowadays, for the modern desk worker, walking and most other physical labor is optional. Convenience food has made eating sugar easier than ever but eating healthy harder. Pain has become something to be masked rather than treated, and these examples only scratch the surface of the underlying issues.

Since you are reading this book, you've already recognized that these are real issues and that detox tea is not the solution—although before we touch on the good stuff, we have to recognize the bad stuff and avoid it.

Ignore unnecessary supplements, fads, and bullshit in general.

Supplements

A supplement is exactly what it sounds like: something you use to help complete your nutrition. If your doctor tells you that you're low on calcium, then please, supplement away. But if your diet is on point, why would you need to supplement it to begin with? I'm sure Milo of Croton, the famous Greek wrestler who carried a calf around the stadium every day until it became a cow, didn't use supplements. He just ate . . . and I imagine cows were lighter back then or the story is total nonsense.

Supplements have massive appeal and have become a $37 billion industry because they are offered as trading dollars for health. Everyone is willing to pay money to lose weight or to get more muscular. What good are your dollars if you don't have your health?

Unfortunately, a supplement cannot live up to its end of the bargain. Sure it can help you achieve 1 percent of your goal, but the other 99 percent is hard work and consistency. A supplement should be used *only* to fill the nutritional gap between your diet or lifestyle and your doctor-recommended nutritional intake.

For instance, if you are trying to gain muscle and aren't consuming enough protein, a protein shake can help you reach your daily goal. If you have an aversion to fish, then supplementing with fish oil isn't such a bad idea. And if you are afraid of the sun or live in a cold place, a little vitamin D can't hurt.

Fads

There are a lot of fad diets out there with a lot of their own branded food that they want to sell to you. It's their business model—SlimFast, Atkins, Jenny Craig, you name it. They all sell *products*. And while, yes, a lot of them do help people, at the end of the day, it's more important for these companies to sell low-calorie candy bars than it is to improve your health and nutrition. The best thing you can do is just eat real food.

Real food is food. It comes from either the ground or animals. We can cook it and combine it in a million different ways to make healthy, delicious meals. There has never been a chocolate bar that was healthier than spinach, and there probably never will be. I hope to God that I'm wrong, but as of 2019, it's a fact.

I'm not preaching the Paleo Diet or trying to convince you that no processed foods can be healthy, but it's a lot easier to just avoid all the crap than it is to sort through all the options to find something good for you. For today, just start increasing the number of foods you consume that aren't made in a factory. Remember that the more times something has been handled or changed from its original form, the more likely it has had unnecessary calories added to it.

Bullshit in General

If you are an internet user who has ever clicked on something related to health or fitness even by accident, there is no doubt you have become inundated with articles titled "The Easiest Way to Lose Weight," or "Get a Six-Pack in Six Weeks."

Here is some of the most common bullshit in the health and fitness industry as of this writing:

BULLSHIT: Fruit is making you fat

TRUTH: Fruit does NOT make you fat. The reason this myth has gained traction lately is because there is fructose (a type of sugar) in fruit. However, if you are getting your fructose from real fruit and high-fructose corn syrup is not a regular part of your diet, you have nothing to worry about.

BULLSHIT: Detoxes of any kind

TRUTH: Your liver and kidneys are what remove the toxins from your body—not a mixture of lemon juice and maple syrup. If you have an urge to do some sort of detox, try intermittent fasting (see chapter 2.3).

BULLSHIT: Women should do lots of reps with light weights to "tone up"

TRUTH: The muscular systems of men and women are essentially identical. Women have some extra fat deposits for baby making and feeding purposes, but the structure of their muscles is indistinguishable from men. The goal of your workout should always be to increase your strength; becoming "too bulky" is the result of a deliberate muscle-building program, not something that happens by accident.

BULLSHIT: You need to constantly eat in order to "stoke your metabolism"
TRUTH: Your metabolism will work no matter what frequency you "stoke it" at—it isn't like a campfire that needs to be tended. Think of it more like a gas tank: on a road trip, you wouldn't want to stop for gas six times a day. Eat when you are hungry, and DON'T eat when you are not.

BULLSHIT: You need to create "muscle confusion" to get strong
TRUTH: Variety is the spice of life, but you don't need to be constantly changing the routine you do. Your muscles adapt to the stress placed upon them; if the stress is always the same, they will stop adapting. However, if you did the same six exercises for years and simply varied the weight, the repetitions, and the tempo, you would never plateau.

There is a lot more bullshit out there that wasn't covered above, and I encourage you to read everything related to health and fitness with an intense skepticism and make it prove that its claims are true—including this book. Most online articles won't include citations, and, if they do, sometimes you'll find they are just links to other articles written by the same person. A lot of "experts" use before-and-after pictures to prove their system works. But a lot of the pictures are taken on the same day and just photo-shopped.

What works in health, fitness, and pain relief isn't sexy. It is a consistent effort, simple daily practices performed over an indefinite period of time, and a focus on diet.

CHAPTER 2

Diet: Choose your own adventure

ONE OF THE BIGGEST PROBLEMS with the diet industry is the refusal to recognize that there is more than one solution to the obesity epidemic. Whether it's veganism, paleo, intermittent fasting, keto, or the newest fad, every diet book or guru touts one strategy as the "end all be all" of diets. They quote their idolized MD's dogma with religious fervor and rarely stop to consider another's point of view.

So let's look at the big picture.

The world is a big place, and many people eat in many different ways. There are diets we've found to be healthy (like the Mediterranean diet) and diets we've found to be unhealthy like (the Western or American diet). Unfortunately, as a consequence of improved technology and globalization, the Western diet has been spreading across continents like Genghis Khan. Wherever the Western diet goes, obesity and heart disease follow.

Doctors, dietitians, and intelligent individuals alike view this epidemic as a bad thing for obvious reasons and have been combating it ever since with an ever-increasing confusion of diets. These diets and lifestyles that were created for the greater good have turned into warring factions that have totally forgotten who the true enemy is. What vegan zealots and paleo partisans no longer recognize is that they are on the same side. They both were created to help people live healthier lives. Certain lifestyles may resonate more with you as an individual: perfect—lean into that.

If you don't like eating meat, don't eat it.

If you think breakfast is a waste of time, skip it.

There is a diet plan that fits your predisposition; there is even a guy who promotes an ice cream diet. You can watch his YouTube videos as he slowly becomes malnourished; it starts off funny but then gets a little sad.

Choosing your own adventure is about recognizing your predilections, not joining a cult. Establish your why and reach *your* goals.

Why diet?

Why limit ourselves? Why not enjoy every moment by scarfing down candy?

In terms of dieting, the most important step is establishing why we are doing it in the first place. Do you want that beach bod? Do you want to decrease your risk of disease? Have more energy? Have better sex? Play with your grandkids?

Eating healthy helps you improve your body composition and look super sexy; it helps you sleep; it reduces your risk of diabetes; it lengthens your life; it improves your mood; and it does the immeasurable: it makes you feel good. Not good as in happier, or good as in stronger, although it is capable of doing both. It makes you feel good as in healthy. The feeling of health is an intangible one that you'll have to experience in order to reference. However, feeling *not* good is something that resonates with everyone.

You should come up with your own reason for improving your diet. In fact, write it down, and stick it to your fridge or pantry to help you stay on track. A healthy diet isn't something you try for a few months and then go back to your usual routine; a healthy diet is how you eat for the rest of your life.

Choose your own adventure, and do what works for you! You don't have to strictly adhere to it every single day, but you must create a framework for yourself in order to have long-term success. A major reason most fad diets fail is that health professionals are trying to fit *your* life into *their* framework. It is *your* life, so *you* need to choose the framework that *you* can live with indefinitely.

> A healthy diet isn't something you try for a few months and then go back to your usual routine; a healthy diet is how you eat for the rest of your life.

Remember that if a program costs money, you are being sold something. These programs make money by preying on people's insecurities. They want you to get fantastic results in an incredibly short amount of time so they can better advertise this success on an infomercial.

That is not to say that there is anything wrong with wanting to quickly lose weight. Seriously, who wouldn't want to lose weight fast? You just need to understand that once you've dropped the weight, you must maintain most of the habits you've adopted to achieve that goal in order to stay at your current weight. Ninety-five percent of diets fail because people regain when the diet "ends." The truth is that the diet can never end, or your weight will yo-yo forever.

The changes must be permanent. Failing to understand this crucial fact has led to the prevalence of cleanses, fads, and otherwise unhealthy or unsustainable diets. Programs based on rapid body transformation have become revered as the gold standard. Their appeal is that they work wonders in the early stages of losing weight.

However, allow me to let you in on a little secret of the strength-and-nutrition world. Every program works at the beginning. Changing your diet in any way that is slightly positive works. In order to achieve long-term success in a fat-loss program, the only thing you have to do is maintain a calorie deficit. There are many ways of achieving that and no one-size-fits-all solution. However, there are a few concrete rules that every fat-loss program needs to follow to be successful. Regardless of your diet strategy, you must do these four things.

1. 50 percent of what you eat should be vegetables

If 50 percent of your diet is vegetables, then at least 50 percent of your diet isn't crap.

Vegetables are the best carbohydrates. I know that carbs have essentially become viewed as weight loss's kryptonite, but think about them like this: There are two main types of carbohydrates—fibrous carbs and starchy carbs. Fibrous carbs are very filling and low in calories; they include foods like broccoli. Starchy carbs, like rice, are probably what you think of when you hear *carbohydrates*. These are also pretty filling but not quite so low-calorie. For example, three cups of broccoli and three cups of brown rice take up the same amount of space in your stomach. You'll feel full after eating either option. However, the broccoli contains about 90 calories, and the brown rice about 650.

Easy action step:
Make 50 percent of your diet vegetables.

*Add vegetables to every meal. Some people struggle to add veggies to breakfast. Try a veggie omelet, a green smoothie, or a breakfast salad.

2. Sleep!

No matter how good you are about your diet and exercise, inadequate sleep will significantly hinder your progress. Sleep helps regulate the hormones that control your metabolism and appetite.

If your appetite increases and your metabolism slows down, you are in trouble. So guard your sleep like the precious commodity it is!

Easy action step:
Get sufficient sleep.

*The average adult needs between six and eight hours.
Find out what you need to function at your best,
and obtain it every night.

3. Stay hydrated

Everyone knows that you should drink water, but a lot of people don't know why. First off, your body is 70 percent water; it makes up a large portion of your blood, organs, and even your bones. Water is necessary to regulate body temperature, transport nutrients, and build muscles; it also plays a role in digestion, respiration, and even reproduction. Water is the most essential nutrient there is. It also happens to be the cheapest and most abundant.

Easy action step:
Start every day with a large glass of water!

*Drinking a big glass of water first thing in the morning
helps you in multiple ways:
• It fills you up.
• It rehydrates you.
• It kick-starts your metabolism for 0 calories.

4. Track your intake

This one isn't a must; not everyone is going to diligently track their intake. However, this is one of the most effective tools for weight loss when starting a strength program. Food diaries are beneficial for weight loss for two reasons: first, because writing down everything you eat makes you conscious of what you consume, like that handful of nuts or those five grapes. This practice takes all your snacks into account.

Second, if your goal is weight loss, you won't want to write down unhealthy entries in your diary, which will make you less likely to eat them. On the other hand, you'll be pretty excited about logging that salad.

The best part of a food diary is that it helps give you a clear picture of the most important thing when it comes to weight loss: calories in versus calories out.

Easy Action step: Create a food diary!

Not only is it the most commonly neglected step, but it also often has the largest impact. On top of that, it's easier than ever nowadays. Multiple free apps on your phone can track your calories and macronutrients for you.

If you do only these four things and skip the rest of the diet information, you already have the framework necessary to achieve a far better diet than the average American. In fact, I've had a few clients who never needed any dietary help beyond these four impactful lifestyle changes.

A specific case that stands out is my client Jim. He came to me with a desire to lose ten pounds for summer. I asked him to do these four things, and he lost five pounds in ten days. He is certainly an outlier, but he hated writing in the food journal so much that he found it easier to eat only three meals, remember all of them, and write them down before the day ended. He said, "I stopped snacking because I didn't want to remember it."

In addition to these four easy steps for your nutrition, I suggest you follow one of these incredibly easy-to-implement diet frameworks: flexible dieting, paleo smart, or intermittent fasting.

It doesn't matter if you are a vegan, a pescatarian, or a carnivore; these frameworks fit all lifestyles. Every living human is an omnivore by definition, regardless of what you choose to put in your body. You have the equipment for digesting plants and meat. Surviving a desk job requires more than just the correct equipment; it requires discipline and a plan for regulating birthday cake intake.

CHAPTER 2.1

Flexible dieting
How to win at eating

Flexible dieting is the concept of adding up all the calories you'll burn in a day and trying to eat less than that number while also maintaining a good macronutrient ratio (carbs/protein/fat). Flexible dieting is one of the best lifestyle choices you can make for getting healthier, because nothing is off-limits. You can eat healthy all day and enjoy a donut for dinner as long as you stay within your calorie allotment and have eaten your veggies and protein for the day. Theoretically, you could eat ice cream every day if you chose (albeit in small quantities). The point is, your favorite foods and alcohol are totally able to be part of a balanced diet.

However, this strategy isn't for everyone. It involves diligently tracking everything you consume and scanning tons of nutrition labels.

This strategy is great for people who:

> Keep detailed records

> Can handle moderation

> Are otherwise organized

How do you do it?

1. Get an estimate of how many calories you burn in a day (Google calorie calculator).

2. Take your body weight and multiply it by 0.6; the result is your target grams of protein per day.

TIPS FOR SUCCESS

1. *Think of calorie allotment in terms of a week, not a day.*

    If you think you'll drink once a week, you'll need to allot calories for that. Drinking is incredibly calorically dense; maybe your new drink will be a vodka water?

   Say you have 14,000 calories for the whole week and plan on going out Friday. Maybe instead of 2,000 calories every day, you go 1,900 calories a day, with 2,700 on Friday. That way you still maintain your calorie-deficit and weight-loss goals.

2. *Get a food scale and some measuring cups.*

    The most common reason calorie counting fails is because people underestimate the amount of food they consume. Measure every serving.

3. *Remember, this lifestyle isn't without its flaws.*

    The number we estimated for your calorie allotment is only that: an estimate. People's resting metabolic rates vary, even among similar sizes and ages. The calories you burn per day can be affected by certain genetic factors, the way your organs function, or even the temperature in the room. That's why it's important to take stock weekly, and if you see no progress after two weeks, subtract one hundred calories from your daily allotment.

Now you have two things to focus on: remaining under your calorie allotment and hitting your grams of protein in the day. That's it. Do it, and you will lose weight.

The amount you go under your calorie allotment will determine the speed of weight loss. I suggest a *small* calorie deficit of one hundred to two hundred calories. When it comes to flexible dieting, slow and steady wins the race. We are trying to establish a new norm for you, not three days of extreme dieting followed by a week of binging and feeling bad about yourself. Remember, the best diet is the one you can stick to indefinitely.

CHAPTER 2.2

Paleo Smart
Nonprocessed foods and decreased insulin resistance

One of the most popular diet trends in America is the paleo diet, based on the idea that you should eat only food found in the Paleolithic age. The paleo lifestyle has gained a lot of traction as of late, because it's effective, easy to follow, and generally healthy. This plan is called Paleo Smart because paleo is an effective diet plan, but the logic behind adhering to it isn't that solid.

Essentially, it says, "Let's do what our ancestors did, because they were healthy." But the Paleolithic era was so long ago that we have a tenuous grasp of what their health and day-to-day lives were actually like. We know they didn't eat bread, because it didn't exist; neither did coffee, toothpaste, or amoxicillin, yet the latter are all considered paleo. Paleo Smart has nothing to do with your ancestors and everything to do with what you put in your body.

The reason people love this plan is because it has fewer guidelines and almost no measuring—besides, it's hard to overeat vegetables. The rules are simple: if it comes from the ground or an animal, you can eat it. No processed foods. Nothing that comes in a box.

Paleo also has praise heaped upon it because of the obesity epidemic. There are two main reasons for the prevalence of obesity. The first and primary cause is excessive calorie consumption, which is why all weight-loss programs call for a decrease in overall calories consumed. The secondary culprit is insulin resistance. Insulin is what tells the cells in your body to grab the sugar out of your bloodstream and use it for energy after a meal. Insulin resistance is essentially when your cells stop taking insulin's calls, because the constant calling annoys them. If this continues, your blood sugar will rise, and you could develop type 2 diabetes. Because the paleo diet cuts out processed food, it removes all processed sugar and high-fructose corn syrup from your diet. This results in much less insulin being constantly released to process the sugar and thus less likelihood of developing insulin resistance.

However, paleo also gets a lot of flak because it's not necessarily a guarantor of weight loss. You can absolutely *gain* weight on this diet—potatoes, nuts, and animal fats are all calorically dense. But if you follow step one to a healthy lifestyle and eat veggies for half your food intake, you shouldn't have too much of an issue with maintaining a calorie deficit.

Another common gripe with paleo is that you'd be hard-pressed to find fruits and veggies that look anything like their Paleolithic predecessors. Have you seen the size of apples lately? This is a trivial complaint that can be totally ignored.

Another source of ire among critics is the host of "paleo products," such as cookies or pasta made with all-natural ingredients. To be honest, that criticism is justified—these are simply marketing companies trying to make money and should be ignored.

This strategy is great for people who:

> Like easy-to-remember rules

> Hate tracking food intake

> Prefer absolutes to moderation

How do you do it?

1. Eat only things that come from the ground or animals.

2. Avoid processed foods, sugar, and high-fructose corn syrup.

There are two very controversial issues in the paleo community. The first is dairy. Most anthropologists agree it wasn't consumed

TIPS FOR SUCCESS

1. *Plan a cheat meal.*

    Nobody is perfect forever; cheat on your terms. It's better to plan to have a cheat meal once a week and look forward to it than accidentally eat an entire pint of Ben and Jerry's because work sucked.

2. *Plan your snacks.*

    Eating paleo at restaurants is easier than you think—it is hard to find a place that doesn't have salad on the menu nowadays. Plus it's 2019, so just tell people you are gluten intolerant, and they'll make a dish "paleo" for you. Snacks are more difficult, though. You can't get fresh fruits and veggies everywhere, but you can bring them with you from home.

3. *Don't panic.*

    If your weight goes up instead of down, increase your leafy vegetable consumption, and decrease everything else. This will always work.

4. *Avoid fake paleo.*

    Granola, most yogurt brands, and most trail mixes try to market themselves as healthy and all-natural. They usually aren't.

5. *Make exceptions, but not too many.*

 Condiments are the hardest part of the paleo diet. If you need ranch dressing to eat salad, then have it, but be sure to measure out a serving. Remember, the goal of every diet is just to do better than the day before.

in the Paleolithic era, so the diehard paleo folks are very anti-dairy. And absolutely, you will likely have more weight-loss success excluding dairy, but it isn't essential. Our diet plans are designed for long-term success, and if you enjoy having dairy as a part of your diet, by all means, go for it. Dairy is perfectly healthy; you can eat things like 100-percent organic, no-sugar-added yogurt, or all-natural cottage cheese. Stay away from ice cream and processed cheese, though.

The second controversial issue is alcohol. And similar to dairy, *you will have more weight-loss success excluding alcohol.* But again, this plan should be something you can do indefinitely. If you like to drink, by all means, drink—in moderation. For the record, the most "paleo-approved" choices in that regard are straight vodka and dry white wine, but there's no need to punish yourself. Just think "no soda mixers, and no beer," and try to limit alcohol consumption to once a week.

CHAPTER 2.3

Intermittent Fasting
The subtle mix of self-discipline and gluttony

My personal diet strategy that strays a little from the mainstream but is incredibly effective is known as intermittent fasting. Like other lifestyles (such as paleo), this takes its roots from our primitive ancestors, for whom food was never guaranteed. They would spend their days looking for food and—if they were successful—their evenings feasting on the bounty. Intermittent fasting suggests adopting the same strategy of feast and famine. Of course, we like to focus our energy on the first part, because while fasting is easy, eating right is much harder.

Fasting isn't for everyone, because everyone responds differently to it. I grew up fasting on Yom Kippur, and, as a thirteen-year-old boy, it was the hardest thing I'd ever accomplished in my life. As I've gotten older, I don't notice the fasting until about twenty hours in, and each year it gets easier. This isn't the case for my sister; for her, fasting is still a challenge.

Everyone is different—some people can fast all day without even noticing, while others get grumpy if they don't eat every three hours. The intermittent-fasting strategy is designed to help anyone fast without ever feeling like they are starving.

This diet strategy works because it targets both of our obesity culprits. Most important, it decreases the amount of time per day that you spend eating, which often decreases overall calorie intake. Additionally, the long breaks between feasts can help decrease insulin resistance, our other weight-gain culprit.

As a personal trainer, I had a young woman come to me for weight-loss advice. She was upset because she wasn't seeing results, and her current trainer "made me wake up early to eat breakfast." After simply suggesting she skip breakfast if it didn't bring her joy and change nothing else, as she was already eating a healthy diet, she lost five pounds in five weeks.

This diet strategy is the least popular of those suggested, because most people tend to find it intimidating. But don't fret! It really isn't that hard.

If you choose to adopt this strategy, there is a common myth we should quickly bust.

MYTH: If you choose not to eat, your body goes into "starvation mode" and decreases the calories you burn at rest, making it impossible to lose weight.

TRUTH: If you eat fewer calories, you'll lose weight. If "starvation mode" was a real thing, anorexia would be impossible.

It's true that if your weight is constantly fluctuating, losing weight can become more challenging because, under those conditions, your metabolism can get a little funky in the short term. Time, consistency, and resistance training can offset any of the funky stuff.

This strategy is great for people who:

> Have high levels of self-discipline

> Don't feel hungry in the morning

> Are short on time

> Prefer big meals

How do you do it?

1. Ideally consume nothing but water during your fast. If needed, you can drink coffee or tea but definitely no sweetener.

2. Eat your food for the day in a 9- to 11-hour window. (Most people go from 10 a.m. until 7 p.m., but any window works.)

TIPS FOR SUCCESS

1. *Break your fast with a big salad (and some protein).*

    We still want 50 percent of your diet to consist of vegetables, and this is an easy way not to overeat high-calorie foods immediately following your fast.

2. *Don't binge.*

    Think of this strategy as forced portion control. If you try to eat the same amount of calories in one sitting as you normally eat in a day, you probably won't feel too great.

3. *Keep it in perspective.*

    Remember, half a day without food isn't really the big thing people make it out to be. Don't stuff your face to prepare for your fast. You'll be fine.

4. *Don't eat crap.*

    Just because you fasted for fourteen to sixteen hours, that doesn't give you an excuse to binge on junk food. If you fast and then eat crap, you render the fast meaningless.

If fasting for fifteen hours becomes too challenging, feel free to eat leafy green veggies during that time. At no point should you ever be in extreme discomfort.

Finally, remember you still have to feast on *healthy* foods. Do not use fifteen hours of fasting as an excuse to eat junk. Aim to cut out processed foods, and you'll have no trouble finding success with this strategy.

CHAPTER 2.4

Diet Wrap-Up

All diets have advantages and disadvantages. Again, the most important thing is finding a diet that works with your lifestyle!

Too often, people try to change their lives to fit the rules of the latest diet fad instead of practicing a diet that works with how they already live. Losing weight and eating right isn't as hard as people make it out to be. It's not about abstaining from your favorite foods or never having fun again. All that matters is consistently making those small positive choices, like having water instead of juice or a salad instead of a sandwich.

Seeing results from those small positive choices takes time, though. In general, people overestimate what eating healthy can do for you in a month but *vastly* underestimate what it can accomplish in a year. Remember: *The best diet is the one you can maintain indefinitely.*

If you can do the little things right and avoid any bullshit, healthy-diet "hacks" sold on the Internet, a year from now, you will see significant improvement in your body composition.

More things to avoid:

1. Any diet products

Bars, shakes, and other supplements might not be unhealthy, but they are unnecessary. Most protein bars are simply candy bars with added protein, but, in an emergency, they're still better than the alternative. If you are going to grab a protein bar, make sure there is little to no added sugar and the calories are relatively low. Shakes are a fine way to get some extra protein because they are easy and can be low calorie, but most other supplements (excluding vitamins and fish oil) are just a good way to throw away money.

2. Overeating

It's easy to eat too much healthy food and gain weight. There is nothing wrong with a baked potato and a cup of cashews, but if you eat two of each, you'd have consumed around 1,800 calories. Try to operate under the one-plate rule: have a reasonably sized plate, and fill it only once per meal.

3. An unbalanced diet

Part of eating healthy is a balanced diet. Our diet plans have guidelines that facilitate balanced eating, but you should understand what those portions look like in a meal: a palm of protein, a cupped hand of carbs, and a thumb of fat. Remember to stick to the basics: half of what you eat throughout the day should be vegetables, and you should never feel like you are starving yourself. If you find yourself still hungry after you have your one plate, take a minute, drink some water, and then snack on veggies until you are full.

4. Condiments

What you eat is important, but so is what you flavor your food with. Coffee is a five-calorie drink, but every teaspoon of sugar adds around twenty calories.

Be aware that condiments like ketchup and BBQ sauce also contain a lot of sugars and can hinder weight loss. Instead, try garlic and onion, seasoning blends, steak seasoning, or fresh herbs. Sriracha and mustard are healthier options as well.

5. Carb cycling

Carb cycling is considered a fancy dietary strategy in which sometimes you eat more carbs and sometimes you eat less in an effort to avoid a fat-loss plateau. Carb cycling is an effective diet tool to have in your arsenal, but having a different diet plan for every day of the week can make life a challenge.

Instead, I'd like to introduce a principle called "intuitive carb cycling": on days you exercise or physically exert yourself, eat a larger percentage of carbohydrates, and on days you rest, don't.

For the average dieter, intuitive carb cycling is enough; most people find meticulously tracking the amount of specific macronutrients they eat to be cumbersome. While carb cycling is an effective tool, this is an advanced strategy that isn't necessary for everyone.

Veggies (UNLIMITED)	Protein (PALM)	Carbs (CUPPED HAND)	Fat (TWO THUMBS SIZE)
All leafy green things	Any Fish	Any Fruit	Any Nut
Spinach	Chicken	Potato	Cheese
Broccoli	Turkey	Sweet Potato	Dark Chocolate
Cauliflower	Steak	Zucchini	Peanut Butter
Asparagus	Pork	Corn	Almond Butter
Brussels Sprouts	Eggs	Oatmeal	Cashew Butter
Onion	Egg whites	Pasta	Sunflower Seeds
Cucumber	Crab	Rice	Chia Seeds
Mushrooms	Shrimp	Couscous	Olives
Bell Peppers	Cottage Cheese	Beans	Flaxseed
Green Beans	Greek Yogurt	Lentils	Olive Oil
Peas	Seitan	Cereal	Vegetable Oil
Carrots	Tofu	Bread	Coconut Oil

6. Alcohol

I don't want to be a party pooper, but alcohol isn't doing you any favors. Sure, a glass of red wine for your heart health is totally fine, but when it comes to weight loss, drinking alcohol will sabotage your efforts at every turn. Alcohol is very caloric, and liquor is essentially poison. Don't let anyone tell you otherwise; however magnificent you feel after a few drinks, just remember that if you drink too much, you'll vomit and potentially die.

Besides the fact that we all sip poison from time to time, we should also note that alcohol lowers your inhibitions and increases your appetite. So not only will you initially drink additional calories, but it's likely that, later in the night, you'll also eat additional calories.

Now for the really bad news . . . drinking alcohol can temporarily slow down lipid oxidation—meaning you won't burn fat efficiently while your body is removing alcohol from your system. It doesn't sound that bad, but over time, not burning fat will do more damage than consuming a little extra fat.

So what are we left with?

Giving up alcohol completely is the most effective weight-loss strategy but might not be the most fun. Instead of abstinence, you can try changing your drink to:

1. Vodka, water, lime

2. Gin and soda water

3. Whiskey and water

4. Dry white wine or champagne

This is a lesser-of-the-evils type situation, and I hope you are noticing a theme among the liquor drinks . . . water. Water can bring out the flavor of whiskey and other spirits; however, the characteristic we covet in the water is its zero calories. Not to mention the fringe benefits of water, including helping prevent a hangover, keeping hydration, and helping you stay satiated. Water is the elixir of life; it does everything beneficial and nothing harmful. Consume it whenever possible.

Working your way down the list, you'll notice number four, a dry white wine. Dry white wine is the lowest calorie option in the soft-alcohol category. Beer and wine in general are very caloric, and it takes a few glasses to achieve inebriation. Dry white wine will usually have the lowest sugar content of the wines and the least calories when compared to beer.

If none of the above drinks tickle your fancy, all the better: sticking with water helps you lose weight faster.

If you have read the above and are still thinking, "Well, I can handle this," then here are a few more tips for a fun night out while sticking to your diet as much as possible.

1. Think of calorie consumption in terms of a week, and plan for a binge of 500 to 700 calories. So if you are normally eating 2,000 calories a day, eat 1,900 a day for the week if you know on Friday you are going to rage.

2. Plan your drunk snack; if you know that, once you drink, you are going to eat, plan that meal! It doesn't have to be pizza; you can drunkenly eat cheesy eggs instead.

3. Skip the beer. I personally believe it's the greatest alcoholic beverage ever created; unfortunately, it is also the worst for weight loss, excluding liqueurs and eggnog.

CHAPTER 3

Strength

IF YOU'VE SEEN THE SHOW *NAKED AND AFRAID*, you may be familiar with the concept of a survival score. A survival score is an essentially arbitrary number designed to indicate how well you'll do when left naked in the jungle with a stranger.

The producers of the show rank you from one to ten and seem to base the estimate on past life experiences and attitude. However, once you've seen a few episodes, you quickly realize that not only do they often rank people incorrectly, but they also generally equate their "survival score" with how tough someone looks. For instance, they'll guess a former military man will outperform a hippie chick based purely on bravado.

Regardless of the initial superficial survival score, the contestants stomp off into the wilderness for a week and return with two very different survival scores. It turns out that bravado is far less important than staying calm.

Similarly, when it comes to working out, we may have some preconceived notions as to how athletic we are or how athletic we should be. After a decade in the fitness industry, I can assure you that you don't know how athletic you are unless you work out regularly. When it comes to lifting weights, men tend to assume that they can lift far more weight than they're capable of, and women assume that they can lift far less. I implore you, when starting a strength program, please throw away these preconceived notions. Building strength is about getting a little better than you were the day before. It's not a competition. Where you start is irrelevant; once you get thrown into the jungle, your survival score is going to change drastically.

The first day you decide to work out, take it easy. You are beginning a lifelong journey, and it is best to start out on a good foot. Today is not the day to run a marathon or to lift heavy things. Today is the day to do some basic bodyweight exercises and see where you are.

Does this sound familiar? Billy decides to get back in shape; Billy decides to go for a run; Billy gets hurt and cannot walk for days. Billy decides to give up on exercising for now.

So before we go out on a run, why don't we get an accurate survival score? How well you can complete the basic movements in this section will be a good indication of where you are athletically.

There are basic skills here that you need in just about any athletic activity or to work a desk job without chronic pain (or for surviving in the wilderness, for that matter). The main ones are the ability to pick something up, get off the ground, and squat down.

We aren't going to throw you into the jungle without having you first master the basics. It is dangerous to perform heavy resistance training before mastering the fundamental movements. Too often, when people try to improve their body composition, they begin weightlifting with no guidance. While you probably won't get hurt doing bicep curls every day, you won't get that much stronger, either. If you want to start weightlifting before you finish this chapter, start with farmers' walks. If you can walk with good posture, you can load good posture and do one of the most efficient exercises known to man. To do a farmers' walk, simply grab a weight in each hand and walk, which works your core, your forearms, and your lats. While it may not look like it, farmers' walks are one of the most difficult exercises, and that's why they are a part of every strongman competition.

Strength:
the best reason to exercise

Where to start

Before starting a workout program, the first thing to understand is that body composition is 90 percent diet and 10 percent everything else.

So if your *only* goal is weight loss, focus 90 percent of your effort on your diet and spend at least a half an hour each day walking.

Seriously, if that is your goal, stop reading. Implement a diet strategy and start walking. Come back and finish the book when those two things are ingrained into your daily life.

If you are still with me, let's start by looking at movement through a different lens. Movement means the abilities necessary to be a fully functioning human being, like walking, standing up straight, picking up something safely, and getting off the ground without using your hands.

Movement in general is absolutely necessary in order to help prevent heart disease. It also improves your mood, your sleep, your sex life, and your mental capacity.

Exercise can help all those things, too, but the only reason to create a regimen is to build strength. Exercise is not 100 percent necessary, but movement is. There is a decent chance you'll need to exercise in order to gain the strength to perform some of the movements listed above, although you should remember: the best reason to exercise is to build strength!

Starting to move again after living a predominantly sedentary lifestyle can be dangerous. Yup, I just said moving is dangerous.

Why?

Because there is a good chance your muscles have become too weak to do the type of movements you'd like to attempt.

The best example of this is running.

Remember Billy: someone you know decides his health and fitness are getting away from them, so they sign up for a marathon and start training. Because they're out of shape, the plan is to start at one mile and work upward. No problem, right?

Actually, there are a lot of problems.

First off, a marathon is for elite athletes and experienced runners only. Second, if you haven't been running in years, you shouldn't attempt it out of the blue. Running properly requires a lot of base strength, and going in unprepared is a good way to get hurt. The most common injuries you see in the gym are caused by people running either too much, too soon or with bad form. Both can do a number on your body in the form of shin splints, plantar fasciitis, or meniscus tears.

And yet, most people are still convinced you have to run to get back in shape. You don't. Running is not the most effective form of exercise, nor does it offer any benefit that can't be achieved through a lower-impact activity.

I'm not saying running is bad. If you like to run or play sports, you absolutely should. Just be sure you have the strength to do so without hurting yourself *before* you start.

Check out page 123 for the three strength tests for running. Until you can complete all three, you have no business going for a run.

Since running most likely *isn't* the place for you to start your individual strength journey, what is?

Remember, safety first; the most important part of an exercise program is not getting injured. So, start with our basic movement goals, and build from there.

Let's start with two movement goals that are often overlooked, *walking* and *standing up straight.* People generally think they've got these two covered, but, more likely than not, you have room for improvement.

STANDING UP STRAIGHT—Posture is important; it is one of the first things people notice about you when you meet them. Nonverbal communication is a huge part of how we communicate with each other and with our own subconscious. Depressed people commonly adopt a slumped-over posture, with their shoulders rounded forward and their head forward and down. Does that remind you of what many of us look like at our computer? It should. And interestingly enough, adopting the same body language as a depressed person can subconsciously make you more depressed.

The key to standing up straight is to maintain a neutral spine. For our purposes, let's think of a neutral spine as the posture of Superman. Keep it simple: chest up (*not* all the way up toward the ceiling), chin back, and a slight bracing of your abdomen. Don't suck in your stomach; imagine you are going to get punched in the gut by a toddler, and brace accordingly. Lastly, try to imagine you want to put your shoulder blades in your back pockets; this will cause you to put your shoulders in a better position and release some of the tension in your traps. And voila! You are in the posture of the gods.

Now, all you've got to do is maintain this position whether sitting, standing, or walking your dog until the day you die. Easy, right?

If you are like most people, you struggle to maintain this position for just five minutes.

Here are three exercises to make maintaining your posture easier than ever:

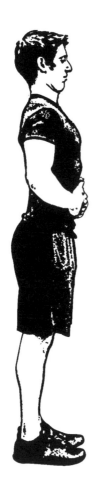 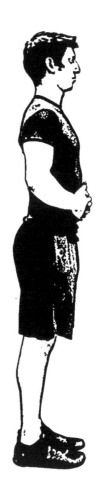

CHICKEN HEADS—While standing up straight, interlace your fingers across your abdomen and attempt to bring your chin as far back as possible. Hold for two seconds, relax, and repeat.

Chicken heads are a great exercise to fight the affliction of forward head posture. It helps you relearn a healthier head position. This motion is tiny but mighty effective.

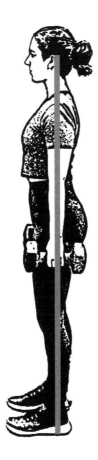

FARMERS' WALKS—Is simply walking with good posture, while working hard to keep the weight you're carrying in line with your body.

The logic behind these is simple. If you can walk around in good posture *with* weight in your hands, you can probably do it easier *without* any added weight. Start with a light dumbbell in each hand, and see if you can walk with them for a minute while maintaining your posture. If so, next time, try a little-bit-heavier weight.

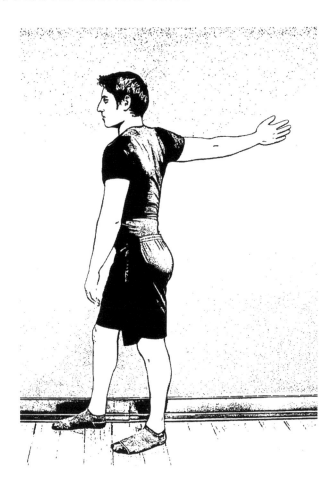

CHEST STRETCH—The more you sit with your shoulders rounded forward, the tighter your chest muscles get. Those tight chest muscles, in turn, exacerbate those rounded shoulders. Therefore, a great step toward better posture is to regularly stretch your chest.

There are a million ways to do this stretch and many different angles at which it will feel good. Everyone has access to a wall throughout the day, so there is no excuse not to try this chest stretch. Place your arm on the wall and turn your body away from the wall. Try it first with your elbow at shoulder height, and you can play around with the angle of your arm to feel the stretch differently.

WALKING—You are probably pretty good at it; you do it all the time. As long as you are not falling forward with every step or letting your head arrive before your feet, our work won't be too strenuous.

Just try to maintain a neutral spine, and keep your feet pointed straight ahead.

If walking with proper alignment is something you feel confident about, head over to the next chapter. But you might find walking correctly to be harder than it sounds.

The most common issue a sedentary person has with walking is keeping his feet straight. If you suffer from this affliction, it is likely a result of one of two things: tight calves or the turning of your hips out or in. This is often referred to as duck walking or being pigeon-toed, respectively. Luckily, both problems have a simple solution.

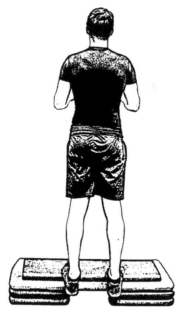

Start by taking off your shoes. Well, whenever possible, take off your shoes. It's like effortless strength training. There are tons of muscles in your feet and ankles that can benefit from some barefoot time. This is especially important, because it is possible that your shoes are exacerbating this foot-alignment situation.

Two steps to improved walking:

Step one: Walk with consciousness; spend more time barefoot.

Step two: Stretch your calves. Simply step onto a stair and let your heels drop below your toes. Try it with your feet straight at first. However, there are two muscles in your calves, and, if you'd like to target one more than the other, you can do so by rotating your foot in or out.

CHAPTER 3.1

Strength: Fundamental movements
Squatting deep enough to defecate

Imagine you are taking a walk in a prairie or a desert, and suddenly you feel a rumble in your tummy. Nature is calling, and she didn't allow a lot of time between her call and her arrival. Faced with two options, you have to make a decision: am I going to go into a deep squat and pretend the prairie is a potty, or am I going to regret the fact that I didn't . . . ?

Most people would choose the former, but to each his own.

If you chose the deep squat, your odds of staying clean are high, but they would be even higher if it's not the first one you've attempted since kindergarten.

There are tons of reasons to squat; it can help relieve tightness in your lower back, you can get out of a chair while holding stuff, and it's one of the major movements that will make your lower body look strong and sexy. However, if the situation arose, you'd be most thankful to be able to hygienically go number two.

Squatting is an easy movement to learn but a tough movement to master.

The reason squatting is easy to learn is because you already practice it about twenty-five times a day without noticing. Every time you sit down or stand up, you are drilling the squat motion. Unfortunately, it is unlikely that you are squatting in a way that activates the correct muscles and benefits your posture.

There is a lot that goes into a good squat, but the two things you need most are mobility and strength. Fortunately, just practicing the squat and attempting to go deeper and deeper while keeping good form will help you develop the necessary mobility and strength in no time.

(However, if you have trouble preventing your feet from turning out or feel restricted in your ankles when trying to squat, the calf stretches from the previous section are the perfect place for you to start.)

How to squat:

Start by standing with your feet shoulder-width apart. Imagine you are going to try to sit in a chair. (In fact, if this is your first time, use a chair.) Maintain a neutral spine, drive your knees out wide, and lower yourself until just before your hips start to turn down.

Keep your feet as straight as possible and flat on the ground. Imagine you are trying to spread the floor apart by creating force in opposing directions. Then, go back up to standing.

To obtain the strength necessary for a good squat, try these exercises:

BOX SQUATS—Box squats are just regular squats with a target. Grab a chair or a bench, and practice standing up and sitting down with great form.

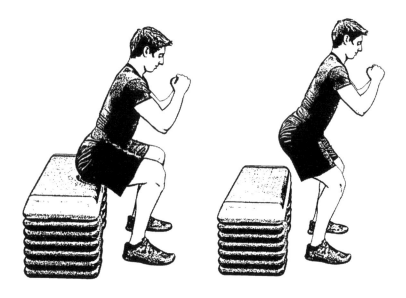

ASSISTED DEEP SQUATS—Squatting deep is hard, and a suspension trainer or simply something to hold onto can help you practice the deep squat. This exercise is a great way to improve your mobility.

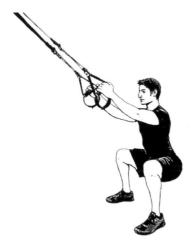

PICK SOMETHING UP SAFELY—The single most important thing you can do for your long-term back health is to learn how to properly pick something up. Hinging properly mobilizes your hamstrings, strengthens your glutes, and helps improve your posture.

Yet, "bending over" is the term largely used when referring to picking something up. When you think of bending, the first thing that comes to mind is taking something straight and misshaping it. When it comes to picking things up, the straight thing we're taking about is your spine. It would be better to just remove that phrase from your vocabulary entirely; from now on, think of picking things up as "hinging." That way, that straight thing, your spine, stays straight.

As opposed to squatting, hinging is hard to learn but easy to master. The basic idea is simple: push your butt as far back as you can while keeping your feet flat on the ground and your spine neutral. However, if you have been spending too much time sitting, this movement will be anything but simple. If you find it challenging to reach the middle of your shin, we've got some work to do.

Once you have the mobility to properly pick something up, you can perform the best exercise there is, the dead lift. The dead lift is the greatest exercise of all time because it is practical, targets a huge muscle group, and makes you look sexy as hell.

The ability to pick things up properly is incredibly important in daily life for obvious reasons. No matter what line of work you're in or whether or not you have children who leave things all over the floor, at some point, you are going to have to pick something up. You don't want to throw your back out while doing it. Dead lifting on a regular basis is the best way to bulletproof your back. The movement strengthens your grip, hamstrings, glutes, lower back, traps, and abs!

PRACTICE THE HINGE MOTION—For the other movements, I gave you some tricks of the trade that have helped many people build the strength and mobility necessary to perform a movement. When it comes to hinging, the only trick of the trade is repetition.

Perform the hinge motion whenever and wherever you have time. The goal is to be able to touch your fingers to just below your mid shin (while maintaining a flat back and keeping your feet flat on the ground).

HOW TO HINGE—Start with your feet hip-width apart. Keep your back flat, and imagine you are trying to push your butt straight back while your shins stay as vertical as possible. When starting off, try standing a foot away from the wall and touching your butt to the wall every repetition.

This leads us to our final fundamental movement:

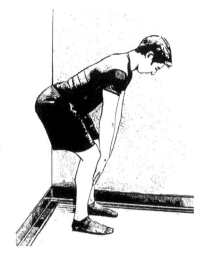

GETTING OFF THE GROUND WITHOUT USING YOUR HANDS; THE LUNGE—You could argue that this is the least important of the major movements, unless, for some reason, you are juggling on the ground; then, suddenly, it's a huge priority. On a more serious note, getting off the ground without using your hands does have practical value. And, as you'll find if you try it, getting off the ground without using the lunge is quite difficult.

Everyone can benefit from the stability, mobility, and strength gained from a lunge. A lunge is the basic movement for athletic performance, and some variation of the movement is necessary for every sport. Plus, Chumbawamba had it right: if you get knocked down, it is nice to be able to get back up again.

The reason this is the last fundamental movement mentioned is because it is the hardest. When lunging, almost all of your weight is on one leg, as opposed to our other movements that evenly distribute the weight between two legs. Additionally, it has one of the largest ranges of motion, as well as the hardest stability challenge. As you are constantly balancing on one leg, this movement takes balance and control to do well.

HOW TO LUNGE—To perform a lunge, start with your feet hip-width apart. Imagine your feet are on railroad tracks, so that your feet always stay in line with your hips, even when they are behind you. Take a big step back, and drop your back knee straight down. Keep your front foot flat on the ground throughout the entire movement.

To get back up, imagine driving all your weight through your front heel, and stand up.

(Don't let your front foot come off the ground; don't let your knee go past your toes to the point it starts to lift your heel.)

For starting strength, you may have noticed we have covered three predominantly lower-body movements. Your lower body holds two thirds of your body weight and a good percentage of your muscle mass. The more muscles you recruit when exercising, the more calories you burn. Therefore, if the biggest muscles are your legs and your core, the biggest-bang-for-your-buck exercises are targeting primarily your lower body.

The most efficient exercises are anything where a heavy weight travels a long distance, the foremost being when a weight starts on the ground and finishes overhead—but let's not get in over our heads (pun intended). We just covered getting off the ground, and we aren't going straight to anything wild. Keep in mind that if a heavy weight moves a great distance from where it starts, it is probably an efficient movement. Just compare the relative movement of a squat to a calf raise, and you can see what I mean. In this example, the weight is your bodyweight. The same applies to upper-body movements, which is great if you wanted more out of this book than the ability to pick things up and get off the ground.

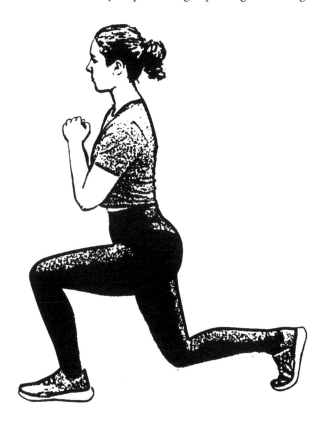

CHAPTER BREAK 3.2

Strength: Upper Body
Train your upper body for a muscular look, lifting heavy things, and opening jars.

When it comes to upper-body movements, contrary to popular belief, there are really only four that matter. In fact, if building a strong upper body were like making a cake, there would be only four ingredients: pushing, overhead pressing, rowing, and pull-ups. Everything else is just frosting and decorations. Just as many kinds of cake can be made with the same few basic ingredients, there are many variations on the four fundamental upper-body movements. For example, pushing could apply to push-ups, dips, or triceps presses. These ingredients are of the highest quality; they use big muscle groups that move a weight the greatest possible distance.

Traditionally, when starting a strength-training program, people want to focus on upper-body movements to give their body a toned look. The way your muscles adapt is based on the weight you train with, the number of repetitions you do, and, in large part, genetics. However, when you start strength training, it really doesn't matter whether or not you want to be toned or bulky or a bodybuilder. You are either building strength and developing your muscles, or you aren't. Building strength and muscle is accomplished through a process known as progressive overload. Simply put, you gradually increase the stress (weight, repetition, intensity/speed), and, if done properly, your body adapts by increasing muscle size, strength, and/or improved oxygen utilization.

This concept is especially important if your weight-training goals are purely aesthetic in nature. When training for aesthetics, there are only two things you need to focus on: building your upper chest, upper back, and shoulders while simultaneously shrinking your waist—aka progressive overload and diet.

That's how all the actors get ready for superhero movies in a matter of months instead of years, and you can do it, too. It's all a desperate effort to increase the ratio of their shoulders to their waist to give the appearance of strength. At first glance, when looking at someone ripped, we subconsciously focus on the inches-difference between their shoulder width and waist width; this is that coveted V-shape. It's the reason most people find the gymnast's body enviable and the strongman's not. It starts with diet, but the next step is pushing weight.

***PUSHING*—SHOULDER PRESSES AND PUSH-UPS**—People generally push incorrectly, and I think that's because people like 90-degree angles. We use them to design everything from tables to rooms to books because we find symmetry attractive—especially T-shapes. I think that fascination is why you see so many people pressing incorrectly.

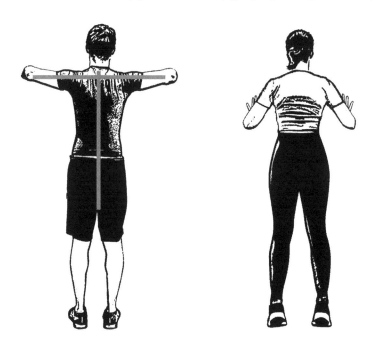

(Incorrect push-up vs. correct push-ups)

In the gym, you often see people doing push-ups and flaring their elbows out to a 90-degree angle, or doing shoulder presses that look more like the YMCA. It's nuts, because those mechanics aren't based on anything anatomical or efficient. People just assume that exercises should look neat and orderly.

The thing is, you are not a table. Your anatomy is structurally sound from all sorts of different angles. When new clients have trouble protecting their shoulders during a push-up or overhead press, I usually walk a little too close to them and ask them to push me back. I've yet to see a client who hasn't immediately adopted perfect pushing form, and I don't think that's because of my body odor. It is because good pushing mechanics are natural.

If you don't have a friend (or enemy) to practice pushing away, you can always lie on the floor face down and attempt a push-up. Or imagine you are trying to push the floor away from you. Without fail, people adopt the perfect press position.

SHOULDER PRESSES—A shoulder press is the king of the upper-body lifts. It moves a weight the maximum possible distance and presents a stabilization challenge for your entire body. A shoulder press is the weight-training equivalent to doing handstand push-ups with the added benefit of *not* having to be upside down.

Unfortunately, shoulder presses aren't the most desk-friendly exercise because they do require some weights. Most bodyweight shoulder-dominant exercises require some sort of inversion, and having all the blood rush to your head isn't fun. When starting out in strength training, you'll want to invest in a pair of dumbbells you can press. If you can press them, they can be used for any of the exercises already mentioned in this book to increase their difficulty.

Just like the push-up, the shoulder-press position isn't composed of neat right angles:

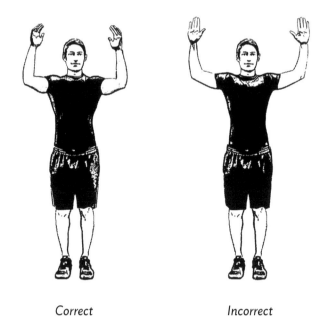

Correct   Incorrect

(In a proper shoulder press, your elbows are slightly in front of your shoulders, not even with them)

PUSH-UPS—If the shoulder press is the king, then the push-up is the prince. This princely activity has the added benefit of requiring no equipment and is doable anywhere at any time. There are hundreds of different push-up variations that can help you build a rock-solid core along with your chest and arms. You can even think of a push-up as a moving plank because that's exactly what it is. In order to do a proper push-up, you must maintain the same tension and posture as a plank throughout the entire movement.

The prince's domain is the office setting, as it essentially designed with a push-up progression in mind. When first attempting a push-up, it can be beneficial to practice on a wall; it is an easy warm up and a great way to dial in on your pushing mechanics.

From there, your desk makes an excellent platform for your next progression. Doing assisted push-ups on the desk or a bench can offer you all the same benefits as the wall except that they are much more difficult.

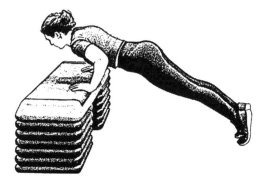

After the wall and the desk, it is time to move to the floor, the real deal. Remember: it is always better to do easier push-ups with good form than harder push-ups with poor mechanics. If you need an intermediary step between the desk and the floor, you can do knee push-ups on the floor.

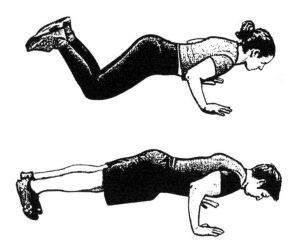

Once you've mastered the floor push-ups, there are many different variations to play with, including putting your feet up on a stable chair and doing an advanced push-up.

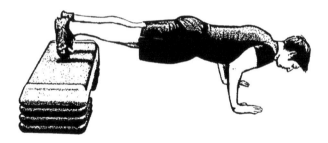

PULLING—ROWING AND PULL-UPS—Pulling offers a unique challenge to the office or home exercise setting. In order to pull, you must have something to pull on. You can push or press against the floor; squat or lunge against gravity; but while you can also pull away from gravity during a pull-up, you still must have something to pull on. Initially, pulling your body weight is going to be very challenging. In order to set ourselves up for success and build a strong base of support for pulling exercises, we will turn to the eccentric portion of the push-up. The eccentric portion of the push-up is the portion when you lower yourself to the ground. It is your pulling muscles that help you lower your chest to the floor in a slow and controlled manner, and extending the amount of time during that lowering phase of the movement can fully change the way this exercise feels.

NEGATIVE PUSH-UPS—Start in a push-up position; lower for five seconds; push back up quickly; immediately begin lowering phase again.

Being able to perform negative push-ups is a good litmus test before attempting harder pulling exercises. However, regardless of your strength, the hardest part about pulling is maintaining your posture.

In general, people have difficulty maintaining good posture, and this is especially true if you ask them to pull something. When you spend eight to ten hours a day sitting behind a desk, it is hard to suddenly adopt proper pulling mechanics as soon as you decide to exercise. In order to pull with good form, you have to do something often referred to as packing your shoulders. Packing, aka setting your shoulders, is essentially engaging the muscles of and around your shoulder girdle, ensuring the muscles bear the load instead of your joints. Think what people look like when they are trying to have good posture: shoulders back and down—the exact opposite of when you are typing on a computer or texting.

The best way to experience packing your shoulders for yourself is to hang from something: a pull-up bar, a sturdy doorframe, or even a bus stop—anything that you can reach above your head. You don't even have to have your feet off the ground to try this. The idea is to effectively shrug while hanging, technically referred to as active to passive hanging. Think of passive hanging as relaxing on the bar, letting your whole body relax, while active hanging involves engaging your shoulders, lats, and core. Practicing packing (or setting) your shoulders is a great exercise in itself.

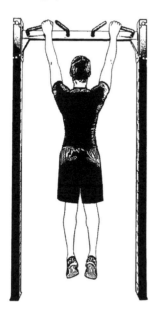 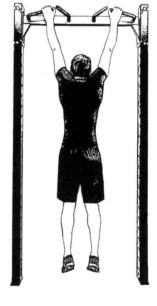

Active Hang   *Dead Hang*

Dead hangs can feel nice as a stretch but are not an effective position from which to begin a pulling motion. The first step in *any* row or pull-up is to set your shoulders.

Pull-ups: Defying gravity is never easy; in fact, it's never harder than when performing a pull-up. Fortunately, the pull-up is the upper-body lift with the biggest return on investment. Not only are pull-ups a great way to build strong, aesthetically pleasing muscle, but the pull-up also has functional value. Have you ever seen an action movie? At one point in every respectable action star's career, they find themselves hanging on to something for dear life, most commonly a windowsill or the edge of the roof, and they always rely on their pull-up strength to get them out of the situation. However common pull-ups are in the movies, we are rarely called on do them in real life. Most Americans older than thirty cannot do a single one, and that is why there is a complete pull-up progression workout in the back of this book. If your goal is to do a pull-up, this little workout program will get you there in no time.

Pull-ups might not be in the cards for everyone's immediate future, as they are highly dependent on your strength-to-weight ratio. Diet is the most influential factor in changing that ratio, followed by strength training.

ROWING—Rowing is to pull-ups as push-ups are to shoulder presses. Rows are the second biggest pulling movement, a core challenge, and a great way to build your sexy back muscles. Rowing is useful in everything from opening doors for elderly people to getting your dog away from a fire hydrant.

The two most basic forms of the row are the TRX (or suspended row) and a dumbbell row. In the former, you are using your body as the weight and the angle you are standing as the difficulty variant. In the latter, it is purely a matter of how much weight you are pulling toward you. In both exercises, you set your shoulders the same way and pull your elbows straight back in order to optimally target your lats and biceps.

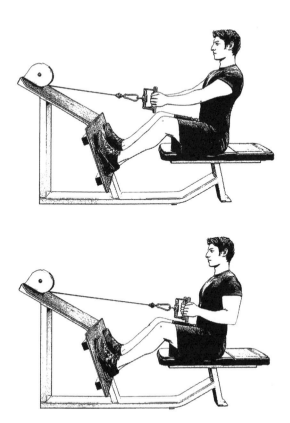

Rows are an effective way to build your biceps without wasting time curling. Both of these exercises can be turned into massive-biceps builders with one little tweak. Pause when your elbows are even with your back; the longer the pause, the greater the biceps burn.

After pushing and pulling, upper-body exercises become a little more about looks than functionality, and there is nothing wrong with that. Targeting little muscle groups is a good way to get that area to visually pop a little more. But remember: if you never did another exercise besides these four pushing and pulling movements, you would still look amazing and have functional strength. More frosting and decoration can be added to the cake, but there wouldn't be a cake worth eating without the basic ingredients.

CHAPTER 3.3
Bodyweight first and tempo

Going into my freshman year of high school, I played summer league soccer; as one of three freshman players, the strength and conditioning was a shock to the system. Imagine just leaving eighth grade with a late start on puberty and stepping into a weight room with bearded eighteen-year-old men preparing for their senior year and training hard in hopes of soccer scholarships.

The first week of summer league was just conditioning, and I could not hang. Soccer conditioning always starts with running drills, and I finished close to last on every one we did. The older kids were literally waiting for me and the other freshmen to finish so they could start the next drill. Later that day, we stepped into the weight room, and the dawdling continued. The first lift we did was the bench press, and I couldn't even move the bar.

After making a career out of strength coaching, I still cannot fathom why the first strength exercise the soccer players learned was the bench press, but nonetheless, I wasn't allowed to try the bench press again until I could do twenty push-ups and ten pull-ups. It made sense to me that I shouldn't be lifting weights if I couldn't move myself. Only years later did I find out that it is simply considered common practice when strength training kids or young adults to start with bodyweight exercises—running, push-ups, pull-ups, and so on.

The concern is that weightlifting could potentially stunt a child's growth, and there is merit to that concern. Strength training can damage a person's body when done poorly at any age, so it stands to reason it could potentially do more damage to an undeveloped body.

Now, I'm not going to tell you that you cannot lift weights until you can do ten pull-ups and twenty push-ups. This is a great criterion for children because they are very adaptable and generally have a better strength-to-weight ratio than adults. However, if you were told as an adult that you couldn't lift weights until you do ten pull-ups, the depressing truth is that some may end up never lifting weights.

We've established some better criteria for an adult: Can you get off the ground without using your hands? Can you do a push-up or assisted push-up pain free?

Nonetheless, it is important to note that weightlifting is not necessary. While I am a huge supporter of lifting weights because it is the most efficient way to improve body composition and build strength, it is not the only way. Bodyweight gymnastics training is also a great strategy for building strength. Just look at Olympic gymnasts; they have some of the best bodies in the world, and they rarely, if ever, pick up a dumbbell. Although it is a bit harder to linearly progress through a bodyweight program than it is to during resistance strength training, with weights, if you can complete an exercise with ease, you add five pounds and try it again. That's why, for certain exercises like the shoulder press, I always recommend dumbbells; with your bodyweight, you can control only two things to vary intensity: volume and the tempo.

Volume's utility is clear: if you can do ten push-ups without breaking a sweat, next time try twelve push-ups. Tempo allows us to have the most creativity; if an exercise ever becomes too easy, try doing it slower. Still too easy? Try adding a pause. The tempo of an exercise can vastly change its difficulty and slightly alter the exercise's benefits.

Every exercise includes three distinct phases of movement: the eccentric phase (lengthening of the muscle), isometric phase (pause at the bottom of the movement), and concentric phase (shortening of the muscle). The purpose of tempo is to ensure that all these things don't happen at once.

FOR EXAMPLE: THE PUSH-UP

ECCENTRIC: Lowering toward the floor
ISOMETRIC: A pause when your nose is two inches from the floor
CONCENTRIC: Pushing up

EXAMPLE TWO: LUNGE

ECCENTRIC: Lowering your back knee toward the floor
ISOMETRIC: Pausing when your back knee is an inch off the
ground
CONCENTRIC: Standing up through the front leg

Where you are with your strength training will dictate the best tempo for you; after a couple of weeks, try a new tempo, and see how the exercise changes.

Note: Tempos are written with the numbers/seconds corresponding to the eccentric-isometric-concentric phases. For example, the classic beginner tempo when applied to a push-up would be read as:

Eccentric (Lower to floor): 4 seconds
Isometric (Pause at the bottom): 1 second
Concentric (Push-up): 1 second

TEMPOS FOR PROGRESS:

The classic beginner: 4-1-1

This is my favorite tempo, and it isn't going away anytime soon. Start with this one. Lowering slowly helps you work on your mechanics, pausing allows you to demonstrate control, and who doesn't want to come up quickly? This is the tempo I use most frequently during my workouts and whenever I teach a client a new lift.

I got this lift down: 3-0-1

This tempo is pretty similar to the classic, the main difference being the lack of a pause. This is by far the most common tempo you'll see in the gym. I prefer to have people go at this pace only once they understand the movement of a specific exercise. You often see people lazily doing reps when they first start out training, and this is not a tempo you should do lazily!

I'm stuck in a rut: 3-2-1

Having trouble improving on a certain workout? Try this tempo. Lowering slowly and pausing for two seconds is hard, so if you're using weights, make sure to use less resistance than normal. The longer pause is awesome for breaking plateaus because it removes the benefit you get from the elasticity of your muscles. Have you ever lowered down for a squat and felt like you just bounced back up? That feeling is the natural tendency and stretch reflexes of your muscles. When pausing at the bottom, you will get no love from the stretch reflex.

Pumped: 2-0-2

Time under tension (TUT) is one of those fitness buzz phrases. Without getting into the sciency stuff, the idea centers around continual work with no rest at the top or bottom of the movement. The key here is fluid movement; you just keep going, never letting your muscles get a second of relief until the set it over. To use this tactic well, program each set for time, anywhere from thirty to ninety seconds. Start with less time, and work your way up. This is an advanced practice for an exercise you are very comfortable with. It's called "Pumped" because that's exactly how your muscles look and feel after performing exercises at this tempo.

You can use vary these tempos along with increased volume to continually improve. The workouts in the back of the book have tempos listed in order to get the most out of each exercise.

CHAPTER 4

Posture and Pain Relief

"SITTING IS THE NEW SMOKING" is the colloquialism of choice when describing the health of our nation. The theory is we are a sitting nation that is doing as much damage to our bodies by sitting as our grandparents did to their lungs by smoking.

Except that is bullshit, and sitting isn't the new smoking.

Smoking and sitting are nothing alike. Smoking is a completely unnatural and slightly strange behavior. Sure we know tobacco, marijuana, and other substances are smokable, but you have to imagine how we gathered that information. It must have been trial and error. The first guy who started smoking surely got some weird looks from his cohorts.

Sitting, on the other hand, is completely natural. If you get tired and need a break but aren't going to sleep, what do you do? If you are hungry and want to eat, sitting is natural.

Sitting is the new smoking only in the sense that you cannot work at a place whose employees are forced to smoke all day long and expect to live as long as people who don't.

No matter how you look at it, sitting in the same position for eight to ten hours is harmful for your body. The problem is not necessarily the sitting itself—it's the chair and the prolonged time in any given position.

As a society, we have landed on sitting upright as the default eating, meeting, and talking position. Sitting can be done in a variety of different positions on different types of seats. While chairs are decent for sitting, since that is the purpose they are designed for, an exercise ball or the floor are preferred and actually offer better protection against pain.

Regardless of what you sit on, eventually you will get tired of the position and need to shift your weight.

Think of it like carrying a case of beer. Carrying something can become really challenging when you do it in the same position for an extended period of time. Yet by changing the ways you carry the case of beer as you walk—at your right side, at your left side, on your shoulder, in both hands, and so on—you can bear the load much longer, more comfortably, and pain free.

Sitting in your office chair is essentially asking your spine to carry the weight of your torso only one way for eight to ten hours. I imagine if you carried the case of beer for eight to ten hours, you'd have chronic pain as well. In order to avoid that chronic pain, we need to go over how to sit.

HOW TO SIT—No matter how much you try to avoid it, at some point, you are going to have to sit. But there are ways of making it less harmful.

If you are sitting in the classic office chair, the most important thing you can do is simply maintain a flat back. Think about having your spine as a straight line from your head to your tailbone. You don't always have to be sitting straight up; you can maintain a neutral spine (flat back) while leaning forward or back. Sitting at the edge of your chair, on an exercise ball, or a stool provides helpful external cues for maintaining these positions. Plus they look the most normal in an office setting.

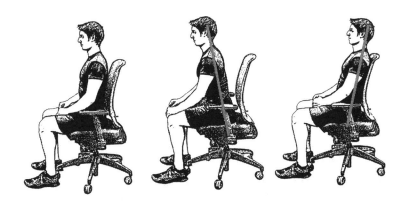

Alternatively, you could sit on the floor in a variety of positions:

CRISS-CROSS APPLESAUCE:

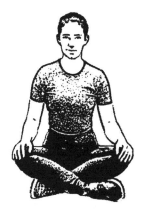 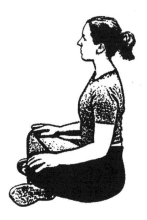

50-50 HIP GLUTE STRETCH:

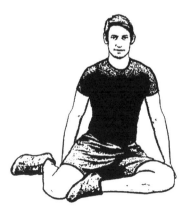

BUTTERFLY:

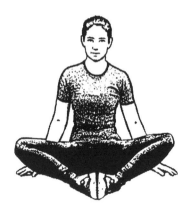

The advantage of sitting on the floor is that you can change positions every few minutes in an effort to avoid getting stiff. The disadvantage is that, unless you work from home and have a coffee table, you'll look like a child.

Regardless of where or how you sit, the most important thing you can do is change positions frequently and take breaks. For every hour you are sitting, you need to do at least ten minutes of walking, standing, or whatever you are into that isn't sitting.

Changing your sitting habits is the first step toward a pain-free life. However, the true campaign against pain starts with posture.

POSTURE—Posture is your first line of defense against chronic pain. It not only prevents pain, but it also influences how your peers perceive you, and good posture can improve your mood.

If you look around nowadays, you may notice that the population's posture has become rubbish. Sitting all day in front of a computer, a television, and a smart phone is ruining the world's posture. Our relationship with these devices strains our relationship with gravity. In the past, when we spent all day walking around and looking straight ahead while hunting, gathering, and being primitive, as opposed to sitting, looking down, and being civilized, we had a certain unspoken agreement with gravity. We will stand as upright as possible in order to move through the world with the greatest ease.

Sticking our heads forward or sitting for too long wasn't part of the agreement.

Remember how when you were a kid, your parents would tell you not to cross your eyes, because if you did it too much, they may get stuck that way?

I'm no expert on eyeballs, but if you spend too much time slouched over, your muscles will get accustomed to the position. Or, in other words, if you have bad posture, you might get stuck that way.

Getting stuck that way would make your life very difficult. Walking, running, and everything else you have to do are just plain harder when you try to work against gravity. You cannot fight gravity; it will bend you to its will and wear you down over time—and it never sleeps.

Have you ever been to a nursing home? That's where the real carnage from nearly a century-old war with gravity can be found. You'll notice that there are plenty of people still fighting the good fight against gravity and walking unassisted. However, you'll see far more people who haven't been so lucky; walkers and canes are as common as hearing aids there. These devices are the result of a lost war of attrition; once someone has become completely dependent on walking with assistance, they have essentially taken one large step toward the grave. I wish I could say that if you don't want to walk with a cane, all you need is good posture, but that's not entirely the case. If you've ever played professional contact sports, any X-games sports, or worn high heels for way too long, you've grabbed a fast pass to the walker store, too.

So while good posture won't necessarily save you from a fate of assisted walking, years of bad posture will guarantee it.

Poor posture is the result of little posture mistakes made every day, at every hour, for years. The more out of whack your posture is, the more stress you are putting on your muscles, joints, and spine. As time passes, the stress becomes worse and worse until you develop some pretty serious side effects; bad posture can exacerbate arthritis, decrease blood circulation, and cause chronic pain.

Chronic pain is also a result of chronic poor mechanics. Your chronic pain is caused primarily by prolonged poor posture at rest and during movement. If you throw your back out putting on your shoes, it probably isn't because you stood up the wrong way one time. It's because you've stood up the wrong way thousands of times and your back can't handle it anymore.

You always hear stories of people throwing out their back picking up a towel or something innocuous. This isn't a result of an extra heavy towel, it is a result of poor movement mechanics over time. Maintain your posture during movement, and you won't have to worry about throwing out your back doing laundry!

One straw didn't break the camel's back because there were millions of straws underneath it. The camel has been picking up straws incorrectly its whole life.

Rounding forward, in particular, puts so much stress on your muscles. Think of your body as a Lego tower. If you have a good foundation and the top of the building is in line with the base, it will stand forever. However, bad posture is like building a Lego staircase to nowhere; eventually, it will just tip over.

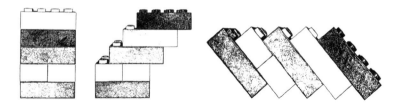

The earlier you correct the chronic mistakes, the easier your battle becomes. The battle with gravity not only affects your body but can seep into other aspects of your life.

Posture influences perception. Think of public speakers you've seen; they don't have to be professionals, just anyone you've seen speak in front of a group of people. The first thing they do is stand up straight and project their voice. Why? Because if you want to be heard, you not only have to *sound* like someone worth listening to, you need to *look* like someone worth listening to.

If someone was giving a speech and they spent the whole time staring at the ground with terrible posture, you would have trouble hearing them regardless of the volume and content of their speech.

When you stand up straight, you project confidence, but when you round your shoulders forward, you look depressed, timid, and fearful. People don't want to hear what you have to say when it looks like you are trying not to be seen.

Not only will your posture change how others view you; it could change how you view yourself.

It has become well established that body language can affect your psychology, from power positions that make you feel confident to smiling to improve your mood. There is a reciprocal-feedback loop between the brain and the body. If your brain says, "I'm happy," your body responds with a smile. If your body smiles, your brain says, "I must be happy about something."

This is awesome when used in a positive manner—for example, Amy Cuddy's TED talk elaborates on the aforementioned power positions. However, it becomes a lot less awesome when you realize that the majority of the population is subconsciously predisposing their minds to depression. Let me explain.

The posture of a depressed person is typically hunched forward, with a rounded back and rounded shoulders. Depressed people subconsciously try to make themselves small and extend their necks forward. The latter is a sign of submission in the animal kingdom, and it doesn't have any redeeming qualities in the realm of people.

Does this posture sound familiar? Look around at the people you see using their phones or working on a laptop. I bet you can spot a number of them with two or more of those depression-posture cues.

So ask yourself, how many hours per day are you adopting this posture? Is it negatively affecting your psychology? Do you find yourself happier when you aren't using technology?

Whatever your answers to those questions, your body will adapt to whatever posture you spend the most time in. If you adopt a depressive posture for eight hours at work, your body will be predisposed to adopting that posture throughout the rest of the day, and your brain might be pushed toward a depressive state as well.

> If you adopt a depressive posture for eight hours at work, your body will be predisposed to adopting that posture throughout the rest of the day, and your brain might be pushed toward a depressive state as well.

CHAPTER BREAK 4.1

Your Feet

Before we get any further into pain relief, sit down, and take your shoes off. Now put your feet flat on the ground and spread out your toes. That's better; we are going to address pain relief from the bottom up, starting with your feet.

People often neglect their feet, yet if your body was a building, your feet would be the foundation. I'm not much of an architect, but without a strong foundation . . . buildings collapse.

Your foot and ankle contain some of the most complex anatomy in the body and are composed of twenty-six bones and thirty-three joints designed to help us balance, maintain posture, and interact with our external environment. Yup, interact with our external environment; they are designed to give feedback to the brain about the terrain, the angle of the ground, and how the body should react accordingly. Putting on socks and shoes is like wearing two layers of gloves and then trying to go about your daily activity as if nothing is wrong. Something is very wrong.

Modern-day footwear is slowly crippling the population. Almost every shoe on the market today comes with an elevated heel and a toe box that allows for little wiggle room. Having your heels raised and narrow-looking feet have no benefit apart from style. It doesn't trick people into thinking you are taller or sleeker; it does, however, tighten your tendons, decrease your ankles' range of motion, and negatively impact the position of your hips, which, in turn, can lead to lower-back pain.

The two biggest offenders are high heels and flip-flops. Both change your natural gait and force your toes to be all scrunched together. If you have ever suffered from plantar fasciitis or any other foot-related pains, I implore you to remove these options from your wardrobe. Gentlemen, don't think you are safe because you never wear high heels or flip-flops; the heel raising and the scrunched-up toes apply to your shoes, too, albeit to a lesser degree.

The best thing you can do for your feet is to be natural. Spend time barefoot, and try to spread your toes apart. There are products that help you do this such as yoga socks and spacers that can be found online. Spreading your toes is important because it increases the circulation through your entire foot. Better circulation in your feet can help relieve symptoms from plantar fasciitis and help prevent future injuries. No matter what, spending time barefoot can help with the health of your feet and ankle and go a long way toward avoiding bunions.

It is important to note that it isn't feasible to instantly transition from a life of elevated heels and scrunched-up toes to the freedom of walking naturally, for a number of reasons:

1. You probably live in a concrete jungle, where the ground is unnaturally hard and unforgiving. Grass has give, even gravel has give, but concrete doesn't give at all. If you go from your nice padded shoes to a minimalist shoe on concrete, the transition will be unpleasant and put you at risk of injury.

2. It's not socially acceptable to be barefoot all the time, and, while minimalist footwear has expanded its market outside of purely fitness wear, they don't look anything like a pair of Hugo Boss. Style is still a factor when dressing for events, and you can definitely find some minimalist casual wear but nothing fancy.

3. Your feet and ankles are weak. The fact of the matter is all this time with your feet imprisoned in unforgiving shoes has left your foot and ankle muscles atrophied. You cannot safely make the transition to minimalist footwear until you build up some strength.

In the shoe game, minimalist footwear is referred to as "zero drop" (a term in reference to the heel drop, which is actually the heel's elevation, but it just means it's flat). A person with strong, healthy feet can grab a pair of zero-drop shoes and start wearing them for a few hours a day. Alternatively, if you have a long-standing relationship with flip-flops and high heels, you can start your transition by grabbing a workout shoe with less elevation. There are plenty of athletic shoes that sport a heel of only four millimeters and can be used as a literal stepping-stone toward your foot health.

*Disclaimer: Please avoid over-cushioned shoes like the plague. I know there are a lot of people who feel better than ever running in their Hokas (which would be considered a maximalist shoe), but it's only because the shoes' thick padding lets you get away with a lot of nonsense. Those types of shoes allow you to run with poor form for much longer before the inevitable injury that results from taking shortcuts.

If you currently suffer from any kind of foot or lower-back pain, I urge you to consider a transition to more natural footwear, as your choice of footwear may be the root of the issue. Some lower-back pain can be resolved within a few days of changing footwear; however, if you currently have foot issues, your path to salvation winds a bit more. I still urge you to consider a transition to minimalist footwear, but it isn't something you can begin while in pain. However, you can begin to mobilize your feet and improve their circulation.

Foot Mobilization at Your Desk

Now that you've made the decision to free your feet from their bonds of oppression, you may find that, in addition to being weak, they are also immobile. Mobilizing your feet isn't as daunting a task as it may sound, because unlike any other stretching, you don't have to even get up to do this. As you already know, I would still suggest getting out of your seat whenever possible, but you can truly do these in a chair during a meeting without anyone being the wiser.

In appropriate work shoes, your feet are in an almost-constant state of dorsi-flexion (toe toward your shin), and sometimes work shoes even limit your range of motion when attempting any other position. Since you've been stuck in that position all day, intentionally stretching the tops of your feet is going to feel great.

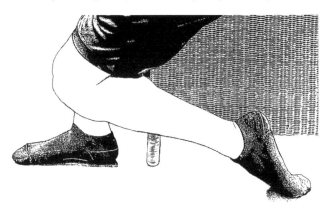

This can be done seated or standing with varying degrees of intensity.

Once we hit the top, we are going to hit the bottom. The best way to mobilize the bottom of your feet and arches is with a golf, tennis, or lacrosse ball. Simply stand or sit with the ball under your foot and work it through the arch and ball of your foot in a slow, methodical way, taking long pauses on points of particular tightness or tension. Hold tight on the tense spots until the tension dissipates.

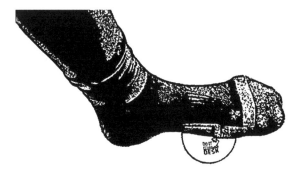

Remember, your feet are your foundation, and, just like a building, you stand the strongest on level ground. Constantly changing the height of your heels changes your stride, and your hips and back have to adjust to compensate for that change. This slight adjustment caused by the height of your heel could be playing a role in your lower-back pain.

CHAPTER 4.2 BACK PAIN

Lower-Back Pain

Back pain is something that affects millions of people on a daily basis. A white-collar worker is four times as likely to go to the doctor with a spinal-related injury as a blue-collar worker. Therefore, it is safer for your back to do manual labor than to sit at a desk all day.

There's just not enough space in this book to include everything we know about lower-back pain and offer a remedy for it. There are plenty of books, therapy programs, and even whole careers dedicated to curing back pain. Our goal in this section is to give you the tools to reduce the pain from any muscular issues as efficiently as possible. If you have pain in your spine, put down this book, and go to a doctor; we are simply going to get your muscular system as healthy as possible and mobilize your spine.

Strength is the most important factor in preventing lower-back pain. But—apart from strength—posture and time spent sitting are the two things you have the most control over. To avoid compromising positions for your back throughout the day, we always want to start by bracing your abs. Earlier in the book, I mentioned that, when you are attempting to maintain a neutral spine while standing, you want to brace like you are going to get punched in the gut by a toddler.

Bracing your abs is like the volume dial on your car stereo; you can turn it up all the way when you want to rock out and lift heavy things. Or you can keep the dial low and do some soft listening when you are just sitting. Additionally, don't forget that you can breathe while bracing no matter what the volume is. You may find yourself holding your breath when you first practice bracing; this is a purely psychological phenomenon. It will take some practice, but soon you will be bracing and breathing at the same time.

How to brace with good posture:

Let's go back to imagining you are going to get punched in the stomach. If you are preparing to lift something heavy, imagine it's Mike Tyson behind that fist. If you are just walking and happen to feel your lower back, imagine instead a toddler or an aggressive teddy bear is throwing the punch.

Do not suck in or try and make yourself look skinny.
That is not a stable position for your spine;
it is a compromising one.

Next, flex your booty; imagine you have a playing card in between your butt checks and you don't want it to fall out. No need to crush the card; just keep it in place.

Pull your shoulders down away from your ears; imagine you are trying to show off your neck.

Lastly, keep your chin back; to help with this you can put two fingers on your chin and gently push back.

Congratulations! You are bracing and are standing with perfect posture; now just try to breathe deeply into your diaphragm.

Another big aspect of preventing lower-back pain is being conscious of how you go about your daily activities—how you stand, walk, and sit—making an effort to spend as little time as possible in a compromising back position (anything but a neutral spine). In addition to having the strength to maintain that neutral spine throughout a host of strength movements, three are going to look very familiar.

THE SQUAT—A great way to loosen up your back.

THE LUNGE—The only known way to get on and off the ground while maintaining a neutral spine.

THE HINGE—The most important movement to master for back health. It teaches proper mechanics for lifting that will save your back.

When we talk about strengthening to prevent lower-back pain, we have to mention bird-dogs. Bird-dogs is the quintessential back exercise and is based around maintaining a neutral spine plus squared shoulders and hips while simultaneously kicking back a leg and pressing out the opposite arm. This exercise reinforces solid hip and shoulder mechanics, builds core strength, and is the complete package in back-pain prevention.

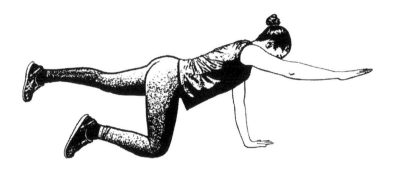

Starting from the quadruped position, hands under shoulders and knees under hips on all fours, extend the opposite arm and leg fully before returning to the start position. Try eight, and repeat on the other side.

Along with strength, we must discuss mobility when it comes to relieving back pain. Having stiff muscles or feeling tight can cause a great deal of discomfort, but mobilizing your back can be done in two easy steps.

CAT/COW—Start on your hands and knees, with your hands under your shoulders and knees under your hips. Look up toward the ceiling, and let your belly fall toward the floor. Move slowly and only within a pain-free range of motion. You now resemble a cow.

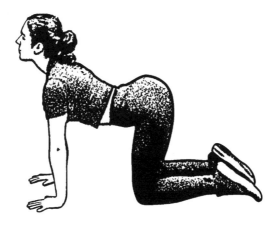

Slowly transition from the cow to the cat position by totally relaxing your neck and letting your head fall between your shoulders, simultaneously trying to bring your shoulder blades toward the ceiling, very catlike. Transition to and from these positions ten times for a single set.

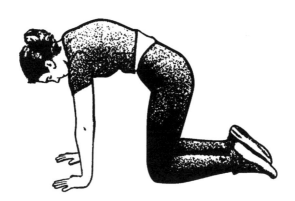

HINGE STRETCH—Just like a dead lift, but we aren't lifting anything, just going through the motions.

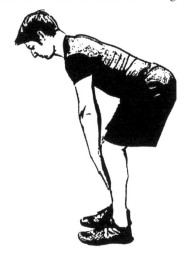

Lastly, before we move on, we have to talk about a fitness buzz-word, glute activation, or, in other words, making sure your butt works. On occasion, lower-back pain can be a result of your butt not pulling its weight. To prevent weak-booty syndrome, try these two exercises:

GLUTE BRIDGES—Start on your back, with your feet on the ground. Raise your hips until there is a straight line from your head to your knees.

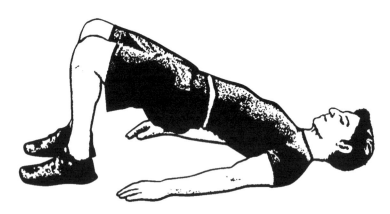

BANDED SIDE SHUFFLES—Start in a quarter squat with your feet hip-width apart. Step laterally, and then bring your trailing foot back to hip distance. Pick up your foot, and put it down. Control the band—don't let the band control you.

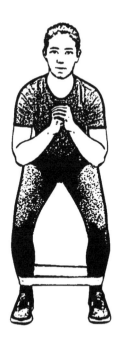 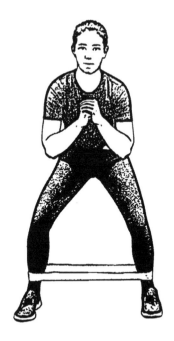

Upper-Back and Neck Pain

Prolonged use of technology causes rounded shoulders and tightness in your upper back and neck. It makes people look like turtles, and, last time I checked, turtles weren't considered one of the sexier animals. It's a condition I like to refer to as "tech neck."

Just like the aforementioned Lego staircase to nowhere, the more forward your head position, the more compromised your spine. It is estimated that every inch forward past normal you hold your head increases the weight placed on your spine and the surrounding muscles by ten pounds. The more time you spend with your head forward, the more your muscles adapt to the new load, and the harder it will be to fix this problem.

Again, when going about relieving pain, we need to strengthen the weak muscles and mobilize the tight muscles. In this case, the muscles that need strengthening are the external rotators of your shoulders, and the muscles that need mobilizing are your chest, traps, and levator scapulae. Think of the external rotators of your shoulders and mobilizing your chest as essentially your anti-rounded-shoulder muscles, while your levator scapulae and trapezius are your anti-raised-up shoulders and tight neck muscles. Nevertheless, all of these exercises are good practice regardless of your specific ailment.

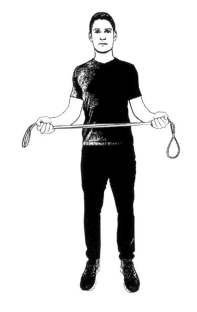

Strengthening your external rotators:

Grab an exercise band or a towel. Hold it with your palms facing the ceiling, and create a 90-degree angle at your elbow. Have your arms hanging naturally; your elbows should be slightly off your body and your hands should be slightly wider than your elbows. Create tension in the band or towel by pulling, and hold this position for thirty seconds.

Mobilizing your upper back and neck:

CHEST STRETCH:

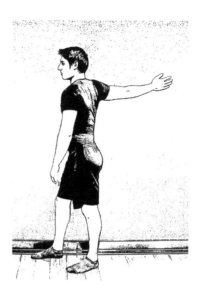

TRAP STRETCH OR MOBILIZE WITH LACROSSE BALL—Stand up straight with your chin back and maintaining your shoulder position; gently pull your ear toward your shoulder.

If the stretch does not provide sufficient relief, the next step would be to try to use a lacrosse ball to get a release. Place the ball on a wall or the floor, and press the body of the muscle into the ball, in this case, the upper trap:

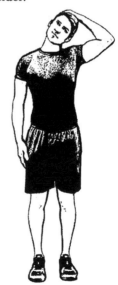

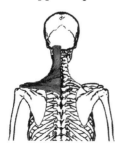

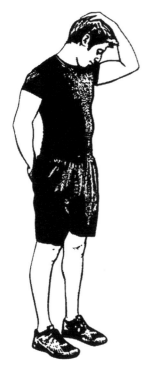

POCKET STRETCH—Stand up straight with your chin back and maintaining your shoulder position; turn your chin toward your front pocket, and gently pull down on the crown of your head.

Unfortunately, there is no quick fix for whatever aches and pains you have from chronic poor mechanics, prolonged use of technology, or sitting too long. Undoing years of bad habits can take months, and it could be a while longer before you get the relief you are looking for. Stick with it; as with your diet, consistency is far more important than intensity. While you could do ten massages, ten ice baths, and ten physical therapy sessions in the next ten days, and probably feel amazing, if you return to your old habits of too much sitting and poor posture, your pain will quickly reappear. Start today; check out the back of the book for a five-minute pain-relief workout based on your symptoms.

If you take nothing else from this chapter to relieve your back and neck pain, take a minute to optimize your workspace.

STEP 1: ALIGN YOUR MONITOR

Sit with good posture at your desk chair and look straight ahead; the very top of your screen should be at eye level.

Make sure you can see everything on the screen clearly so that you don't need to lean forward to read text. Additionally, check to see if you are too close; without leaning forward, try to touch your palm to the screen. That's the closest acceptable distance for most people.

STEP 2: ALIGN YOUR KEYBOARD

Sit with good posture; bend your elbows to a 90-degree angle. That is the perfect height for your keyboard and your mouse. Additionally, avoid using the kickstands available on some keyboards, which force your wrists to bend at an unnatural angle.

STEP 3: PURCHASE THE RIGHT CHAIR (OR HAVE YOUR EMPLOYER BUY IT FOR YOU)

This step is the most important; if you are going to spend hours every day in a chair, make sure it is one that isn't slowly crippling you. Although you are going to strive to sit with a neutral spine at all times, at some point, you are going to relax into your chair, and, when that happens, you need a chair designed or adjusted with your body in mind. Your chair should have decent lumbar support and adjustable height. When sitting in your chair, your feet should reach the ground with ease and, ideally, the seat should not touch the back of your knees.

STEP 4: EXPLORE STANDING OPTIONS

The best way to combat the effects of sitting all day is to sit less. Standing desks are a pricey but effective solution to the sitting problem. Standing allows you more freedom of movement, creates a much easier environment for maintaining a neutral spine, and even burns a few more calories.

However, no matter how well you optimize your workspace, the most important thing is to change positions frequently. Standing the same way for eight hours could give you hip pain just as fast as sitting gives you back pain. Make up an excuse every hour to stretch your legs; your body will thank you for it.

CHAPTER 5

Sleep

WHEN IT COMES TO LIVING a healthy lifestyle, people are always tweaking their diet or exercise routine in order to get just slightly better results. People try cutting out gluten or plunge into the newest expensive workout trend, yet they often neglect the one thing that could have a massive impact on their health and wellness: sleep!

Sleep is one of the most influential factors in your ability to lose fat or gain muscle. Lack of sleep slows your metabolism, negatively influences body composition, and decreases your focus. Basically, lack of sleep makes you fat, sick, weak, and unproductive.

And it turns out you may need more sleep than you think. The average person needs a minimum of seven hours of sleep a night. Everyone's sleep patterns are different, and some people can get away with six to seven hours, while others need as many as nine hours a night. Getting enough sleep helps to prevent illness, regulate metabolism, aid in post-workout muscle recovery, reduce stress, decrease or eliminate caffeine dependency, and function at an optimal level overall.

However, sleeping the appropriate amount is much easier said than done. Modern life makes sleeping harder than ever; the decrease in physical activity and the increase in use of technology makes getting to bed on time and falling asleep a true challenge. Not to mention the added stress of the modern workplace, the ability to binge-watch any TV show at the touch of a button, and the widely used stimulants (like caffeine) that make sleeping feel less of an immediate concern.

If you cannot commit to seven hours of sleep a night, you are unlikely to be successful with a nutrition or strength program. While that statement may appear extreme, it is far from an exaggeration. The reason sleep can be so influential on your body is because of the effect it has on your hormones.

Lack of sleep decreases testosterone and growth-hormone production, and hinders your ability to build muscle.

Lack of sleep can increase your cortisol levels. Cortisol is a hormone you've probably heard referred to as the stress hormone. From a purely physiological standpoint, stress is one of the worst things for your body. When cortisol levels remain elevated long term, you are at an increased risk of depression, digestive issues, headaches, and weight gain. This hormone is so strongly intertwined with sleep and stress that you cannot talk about one without the other.

A lot of people view stress as a psychological issue; they believe stress is something we create in our own lives based on all the responsibilities we take on, our time constraints, and our perspective on how well we think we are doing in life. While lifestyle, genetics, and your mental state play the largest role in stress, your body plays a major role, too.

The kicker is that your body—your posture, your breathing, and the amount of stress hormone released into your blood—all things largely under your control.

Stress is a biological condition; it isn't simply a state of mind. We can use techniques to decrease our physiological symptoms, starting with posture and breathing.

Our bodies influence our minds; if we take sharp, shallow breaths, our bodies react with stress. Think about what happens to people who are having a panic attack.

If we take slow, deep, belly breaths, our bodies react with relaxation. Think about a person sleeping. It should come as no surprise that "take a deep breath" has become more synonymous with calming someone down than holding one's breath.

It stands to reason that if taking deep breaths can help relieve stress when we are panicking, perhaps if we can breathe properly all the time, we can reduce our stress along with it at all times.

HOW TO BREATHE:

Belly breathing or diaphragmatic breathing is the optimal way to breathe. Breathe into your stomach and not your chest.

A great way to practice proper breathing is to lie flat on your back on the floor. Grab two lightweight items; place one on your chest and one on your belly. Relax and breathe, and move only the item on your stomach.

This is how you should breathe both when weightlifting and just whenever you are conscious. Practice diaphragmatic breathing when driving or any time you have a second, and, eventually, it will become second nature. It will turn into your default breath pattern, and you'll be far better off because of it.

The next tactic for decreasing stress will be no surprise for an attentive reader such as yourself. By now, you may have noticed that this health-and-wellness book has a lot of good things to say about exercise. In this case, it's cardiovascular exercise.

Cardio can decrease cortisol levels in the body and increase all the happy hormones like dopamine, serotonin, and noradrenaline. Steady-state cardio is also helpful for improving the quality of your sleep. Just think about how you treat children if you want them to sleep soundly—you just run them around a bit to get 'em all tuckered out. As adults, we sometimes forget how simple it can be. Even low-intensity exercise can decrease circulating cortisol levels, thus decreasing stress, and help you sleep easier, starting a cycle of positive behavior.

CHAPTER 6

Diet, stress, and sleep are all linked

WHEN RESEARCHING THIS BOOK, I was hoping to create a stress-relieving diet, which I thought would be perfect for busy people who want to be healthier. Unfortunately, there is little evidence that foods can help reduce stress, with the exception of warm, calming drinks such as certain teas or broth.

I believe that the calming effects of these beverages are largely unrelated to the actual makeup of the food and more related to the act of indulging in a warm beverage. When you drink something warm, you are forced to wait, take a beat, and let the drink cool. You cannot rush drinking a hot cup of tea. This gives you a few minutes to relax and still count it as your lunch break, which may yield a bit of stress relief.

You can find an infinite number of articles online about foods that reduce stress, but there is no strong evidence either way about this. The articles commonly list complex carbohydrates, anything with antioxidants, fish, and vegetables. While the evidence may be lacking, I wholeheartedly support their efforts to trick people into eating healthier foods like these. In all likelihood, these healthy foods probably do relieve stress, but more scientific research is needed to discover the mechanism.

Although the positive relationship between diet and stress is a little murky, the negative relationship is crystal clear. Stress can cause you to gain weight, from inhaling a tub of Ben and Jerry's after a breakup to mindlessly eating while watching your favorite sports team in the playoffs.

However, what's more interesting is that your psychological state can directly influence your ability to lose weight through a calorie deficit, meaning you can eat a healthy diet and lose weight less quickly if you are stressed. Eventually, you will lose weight, as long as you create and maintain a calorie deficit, but your stress level can greatly influence the speed. That is crazy!

AVOID THE VORTEX

Stress can be caused by any number of things, but let's start by imagining you slept for only two hours last night, and you are worried because you have a meeting that could determine your financial future. Your body's cortisol levels are already raised because of the lack of sleep and your nerves. In order to make yourself feel better, you run out and grab some coffee and a bite to eat. You are in a rush because you want to get to the office early to prepare, and the only thing appealing at the coffee shop is a donut. You go to work, have your meeting, and after work, you decide to go out and celebrate that you are done with that project. You are now pre-disposed to eating a big meal because your blood-sugar levels have dropped since that donut, and you've been stressing out for days.

When most people are stressed out, they search out and eat comfort food. Since comfort food is largely fried and sugary, it should come as no surprise that it will have a detrimental effect on your body. Changes in body composition generally cause stress in otherwise healthy individuals. Stress increases cortisol levels, increased cortisol levels increase appetite, increased appetite causes more overindulging, and the cycle continues. If you are not careful, you'll get caught in the vortex.

THE CYCLE STARTS WITH SLEEP

Lack of sleep increases cortisol, cortisol makes you eat, eating makes you stressed about dieting, stressing makes you eat more. And then—bam!—you're fat.

OK, so maybe it's not quite that simple. Nobody has ever stayed up all night once and, as a result, become fat. If you take one step off the road, you don't end up in a new place; it takes a lot of steps to get there. Stressing about diet choices is a huge problem, as it can actually make you more stressed. Stressing about stress can make you stressed. Stop the madness!

Three steps to relieving stress: Get to bed on time. Do some cardiovascular exercise. Take deep breaths.

I recommend implementing a bedtime for yourself. Odds are you hated it as a kid, but it's just as vital now as it was back then. My clients often find this to be one of the most useful life changes.

Whenever I feel like I'm starting to lose control over my own life, the most important thing I can ask myself is whether I got enough sleep. It can be the answer to a lot of questions: Why do I need coffee every day? Why am I sick? Why am I struggling with simple problems?

Although it should have been obvious, someone had to tell me to implement a bedtime before I actually made a change. So now, I am telling you. Don't get me wrong, of course. A healthy sleep schedule doesn't mean the absence of fun; I'm not suggesting that you get to bed by 10 p.m. every weekend. But, before every work night, get to bed at an hour that provides the sleep you need.

Do you know how many hours you need? Unless you know the extent to which your physiological and psychological needs determine your ideal sleep time, the best way to find out is through trial and error. Grab a pen and paper, because we are going to record some stats.

Pick the number of hours of sleep you think is good for you, and sleep that long for three days in a row, with no exceptions. Keep your diet consistent, and, ideally, avoid caffeine, unless you are already dependent on the morning cup of joe. If you are, keep it in the experiment, or all you will notice is withdrawal symptoms. On the third day, track everything: how you feel when you wake up, if you feel groggy throughout the day, and how tired you are at the end of the day. Keep in mind that this is all relative to how you normally feel.

To find the perfect amount of sleep, you must "know thyself," and a journal is the best way. The reason we stay consistent for three days before tracking is to ensure that your body actually is running on the amount of sleep you chose. If grogginess is still a problem after the first round, add more sleep. Keep increasing sleep per day until find your sweet spot.

DO SOME CARDIOVASCULAR EXERCISE

Cardiovascular exercise improves your mood, reduces stress, helps you sleep, improves body composition, increases your attention span, and helps prevent dementia.

So, what is the absolute minimum you can exercise and still receive all the benefits?

The answer is thirty minutes a day of moderate exercise. Everything counts, even just fast walking. The effect it will have on all aspects of your life is noticeable and substantial.

TAKE DEEP BREATHS

You don't need to sit in a loincloth on your floor and say OHM for thirty minutes, but a few minutes of quite reflection every day won't hurt.

Additionally, one of the only methods proven to increase happiness is to be more grateful. Practicing gratitude is a muscle you can exercise anywhere and any time. Try to think of three things you are grateful for every day; it is a tried-and-true way to make you less stressed and a little happier.

If gratitude is difficult for you to come by, remember that there is always someone out there who has it way worse than you. You have a roof, food, and a phenomenal book in hand for a great wellness read.

Don't let stress control your life. Sleep well, eat well, live well.

CHAPTER 7

Health Hacks

NOWADAYS YOU HEAR about health hacking, life hacking, diet hacking; one thing is for sure—there is a lot of "hacking" going on without a lot of results.

Rarely does one single habit change your life. Those articles you see online featuring the one food that is missing from your diet, the one supplement to boost your metabolism, or the single greatest workout routine are click bait.

When one of your friends says, "Taking fish oil changed my life," it may be interesting to inquire more deeply into the other changes in their lives. Did they change their diet? Start exercising? Change their water consumption? When someone goes so far as to start supplementing, it's generally not the only step they're taking to improve their health. Usually, what changed their life is an accumulation of good habits over time, but the credit goes to their most recent change or the most difficult habit for them to maintain.

Life hacks, diet hacks, and fad workouts operate under the assumption you have a deficiency: fix that deficiency, you'll feel way better after—now may we have some money, please? All of these deficiencies can be fixed through proper diet, exercise, and sleep.

That said, there are some crazy hacks that can supplement diet, exercise, and sleep that aren't total nonsense. Some of the claims of these hacks have anecdotal evidence, but all have at least one scientifically backed claim. Nothing on this list is necessary, but they are fun ideas that don't involve sticking butter into your coffee, drinking vinegar, or the next weird thing that pops up as health advice.

Hacks:

1. Taking Vitamins and Supplements

In general, supplements are largely unnecessary. When compared to real food, their absorption rate is abysmal. A balanced, healthy diet can supply sufficient nutrients to render supplements superfluous. However, if you have an unbalanced diet, a vitamin or micronutrient deficiency, supplements could be what you need.

Fish Oil: This is the only supplement that doesn't use scare tactics to make you take it. We aren't particularly worried about chronic fish-oil deficiency because I just made that up. Fish oil is consumed for the omega-3 fatty acids, but those can be found in foods other than fish. Fish oil is simply the easiest way to get a high quantity.

The list of benefits of omega-3 fatty acids is long. It can help improve everything from your mood to your eye health. It has preventative benefits and restorative properties. Omega-3s can also help decrease inflammation, which is critical for treating arthritis and asthma. Supplementing with fish oil is a good way to get a lot of the stuff really easily.

Vitamin D: In the corporate world, people see the sun less and less. Lunch in the working world generally contains more bread than fatty fish and no time in the great outdoors. Unfortunately, this can lead to vitamin D deficiency, which is the scariest of the deficiencies, as the symptoms include depression, hair loss, decreased immune system, and muscle pain. Instead of supplementing with vitamin D, first try going outside during lunch and eating some spinach, but if you cannot get it naturally, a vitamin D supplement won't hurt.

Protein: In this day and age, it is hard to be protein deficient. As a society, we stress the importance of eating protein for growing big and strong. No matter what your diet is, it is possible to get sufficient protein. Unfortunately, you do still see the occasional person whose diet consists of pizza, pasta, and bread, who looks tired and has thinning hair. Protein deficiency is a scary thing, and if you aren't a carnivore or a fan of dairy, beans, or legumes, supplements are a great option for you. There are plenty of protein powders available that will meet whatever ethical or dietary guidelines you adhere to.

Calcium and Iron: It is possible to get sufficient calcium and iron through a well-rounded diet. However, in an effort to prevent osteoporosis, calcium and iron supplements are a good idea. Osteoporosis is most common in post-menopausal women, so, if you fall into that category, it may be a good idea to get a blood test and supplement if necessary. Nobody wants brittle bones.

2. The Ketogenic Diet

The Ketogenic diet is mentioned here under health hacks instead of in the diet section of the book because it is a little crazy, and most people can't do it. The Ketogenic diet is a high-fat, almost-no-carbohydrate diet. It operates under the idea that utilizing ketones, the fuel source that is created when your body breaks down fat when there isn't sufficient glucose in the body for fuel, improves energy levels and mental function. Whether or not that is a result of utilizing ketones as fuel or simply a result of changing to a healthy diet is not scientifically proven.

The Ketogenic diet, aka Keto for short, is one of the most effective diet plans known to man. It has been shown to be great for performance when it comes to endurance exercise; it greatly improves symptoms of juvenile epilepsy and is good for weight loss. It catches a lot of flack because people try it for a few weeks, don't see major changes, and give up. This is a diet that takes three to four months to truly acclimate to and appreciate the benefits. However, the major problem is that, in order to sincerely utilize fat as fuel and stay in ketosis, you can't really cheat on the diet. Any slip-ups can set you way back. If you commit to Keto, eating a carbohydrate-rich "cheat" meal might initially make you feel sick, and it will even take a couple days to reintroduce them to your diet.

I don't recommend the ketogenic because it is so hard to adhere to, but if you have an iron will, then, by all means, give it a try, and may the Force be with you.

3. Crickets

This one isn't so much a health hack as much as an up-and-coming trend. Regardless of your feelings about eating bugs, crickets are going to be seen more and more in the culinary arts. Currently, crickets are a dietary staple of two billion people, from Africa and Asia to Latin America. Crickets are inexpensive, earthy flavored, and nutrient dense.

Crickets are a great source of protein and are a better source of iron than beef, and they have a low impact on the ecosystem. Humanity's current beef consumption is unsustainable long term; at some point, we won't be able to supply the water necessary to feed the cows. Not only does a cow raised for slaughter drink around 1,500 gallons of water over its lifetime, there is also water used for the crops raised to feed cattle. The amount of water used for raising those crops is immeasurable, but, to put it in perspective:

"If all the grain currently fed to livestock in the United States were consumed directly by people, the number of people who could be fed would be nearly 800 million," according to David Pimentel, professor of ecology in Cornell University's College of Agriculture and Life Sciences.

Nearly three times the amount of people in the United States; a little messed up, right?

You don't need to start eating crickets today, but in the future, when it becomes expensive to eat meat, it might be nice to have already become accustomed to the taste.

4. Cold Therapy

Take a few deep breaths and get ready, because this is going to suck. Cold therapy—cold showers, ice baths, and cryotherapy— all great strategies for relieving arthritis pain, burning a little fat, and feeling good.

Taking a cold shower is the worst; it's no secret. Unfortunately, like eating your veggies, it is good for you.

There are two types of fat, white and brown. Think white fat, heart attack; brown fat, thermogenic effect. Brown fat is used to burn calories in order to generate heat. It is considered brown because when you look at the fat cell under the microscope and it is filled with mitochondria, it has a darker color. Mitochondria are the powerhouses of a cell, and they burn calories to create heat. In theory, with consistent cold therapy, it can turn white fat into brown fat, which is kind of a big deal when it comes to weight loss.

Cryotherapy, in particular, makes you feel awesome because it is stimulating your fight-or-flight response. Cryotherapy puts you in an environment that is insanely cold, which is why you cannot be at all wet when going in or faint of heart. When the temperature starts to drop, your body is thinking, *Holy crap, we are going to die,* and releases adrenaline, which, in turn, makes you feel great, like you just cheated death.

5. The Sauna

It seems as though there are benefits to throwing humans into extremes. Frequent sauna usage has recently been shown to decrease all-cause mortality pretty significantly. Haven't you ever wondered why there are so many old people in the sauna?

It could be because in addition to reducing your risk of all-cause mortality, it also reduces your chance of a sudden cardiac death and cardiovascular disease. The reason this is featured in the health hacks section is because it has become commonplace to advertise the newest spa treatment that will save your life. There are experts all over the place touting the detoxing affects of infrared sauna, or why the steam room is superior, when, in fact, the only mechanism of relevance is the time spent in extreme heat. More research needs to be done as to which heating mechanism is ideal, due to the fact they all use a different means to raise your body temperature. A traditional sauna uses a glorified oven, a steam room uses steam, and an infrared sauna uses infrared to heat you. However, the sauna is the hottest room of the three, and, as of right now, we have research showing that it works.

6. Grass-Fed Beef, Eating Local

You are what you eat, right? You've been hearing that little proverb since you were a child, and there is a fair amount of truth to it.

If you eat too many sweets, you become overweight and have a more ravenous sweet tooth. If you eat a healthy vegan diet, you build very lean-looking muscle.

So when it comes to your beef, would you want it to have been living in a pile of manure with thousands of other cows, sickly, antibiotic filled, and force fed corn mixed with literally any byproduct the food industry considers edible?

Instead, your cow could have been chilling on a field, eating green grass.

In theory, grass-fed beef has fewer calories and more omega-3s, and it is less likely to cause you harm. They are just healthier cows. The only real downside to locally raised cows is the price point; locally raised food is expensive, but, to make it more reasonable, you can buy in bulk.

If money isn't an issue, you shouldn't skimp on this.

CHAPTER 8

Mental-Health Strategies

WHEN IT COMES TO REACHING your health goals, your mind is just as important as your body . . . if not more so.

The way you think about diet and exercise is the key to maintaining a routine in perpetuity. From now on, eating healthy and moving every day is just a part of your life, like brushing your teeth. You wouldn't go a week without brushing your teeth, would you?

We have corrupted our language when it comes to eating right and movement. Most people think of a "diet" as a temporary restriction on delicious sugary food, as opposed to the original definition of the word, which is, "The kinds of food that a person, animal, or community habitually eats" (*Oxford English Dictionary*). Our diets are made up of what we continually eat, not a limit on tasty treats.

The same goes for our language referring to movement. The human body needs to regularly move to be healthy, yet we refer to that habit as "exercise." "Exercise" is a word that generally has a very prescription-y feel to it. "Do you want to walk to the beach?" sounds like a more exciting proposition than, "Do you want to walk two miles at a sustained pace of 3.5 miles per hour?" Both fit the definition of exercise: "Activity requiring physical effort, carried out to sustain or improve health and fitness" (*Oxford English Dictionary*). But one sounds far more enjoyable than the other.

Working out is supposed to be fun; it can be challenging, and there are a lot of days you won't feel like doing it, but it should generally be enjoyable. If you hate working out, you just haven't found the right activity yet. There is a new exercise fad every day, and one of them will tickle your fancy. Do you want to do yoga with goats? Swim with mermaid fins? Run and drink beer? There is a community out there for you. You *have* to do some physical activity to sustain or improve your health. Make it something you enjoy. It still counts as exercise.

Now that we have our definitions in order, lean back on that leather couch, and let's get down to the root of your issues: your upbringing. Your relationship with food and movement have a lot to do with your upbringing. It's not your parents' or teachers' fault; everyone was trying their best. However, there are plenty of habits from your past that may not be benefiting you now. Your elementary school was trying to save money, not provide the highest-quality food available. They taught you a food pyramid that was misguided and never apologized for its inaccuracy. That upbringing sullied the way you look at every meal of the day. Now we are going to identify the problem and, hopefully, eliminate it.

BREAKFAST:

The food pyramid left a generation of people believing that the basis of a healthy diet is bread, cereal, and other carbohydrates. As a result, kids grew up eating cereal, Eggo waffles, and Pop-Tarts for breakfast every morning . . . and loving it. If you can relate to this, we've got some work to do.

All those foods are delicious, but people ate those things for breakfast because the world was under the assumption that (1) they provide the energy you need for the day, and (2) the morning is the best time to eat carbohydrates. Granted, back then, most of the nutrition information came from Wheaties commercials and Tony the Tiger, but this is still a common way of thinking.

It took a long time for people to realize that Tony lied. Not only are Frosted Flakes not grrrreat, they also shouldn't count as breakfast food. Cornflakes covered in sugar fall into the dessert category.

Contrary to the food pyramid, the basis of a healthy diet is vegetables, and they make up a far-healthier breakfast. No matter what your health goals are, you want to start your day off right. You were probably told growing up that "breakfast is the most important meal of the day," and I'd agree with that statement, but it doesn't matter what time of day you eat it.

If you are someone who prefers to skip breakfast and head straight to work in the morning, that's great; just make sure the first meal you eat is something quality. Skipping breakfast is not an excuse to have a donut at 11 a.m. because it's Sally's birthday, and birthdays come around only once a year. Start your day off on a good note; vegetable omelets, oatmeal, or a breakfast salad are all options that put your best foot forward.

LUNCH:

Growing up in the north suburbs of Chicago, Friday's school lunch would consist of pizza with a breadstick, a cookie, and chocolate milk. I loved those lunches, but it should come as no surprise that so did childhood-obesity rates. In Illinois, pizza is considered a vegetable because of the tomato sauce. Despite the fact that pizza is obviously not a vegetable, it should also be noted that tomatoes are actually fruits. They are considered vegetables only in America because the Supreme Court ruled that they are used in the culinary arts as a vegetable and should have a tariff to match.

Regardless of how you look at a tomato, pizza is no vegetable, and school lunches are notoriously unhealthy. Pizza, grilled cheese, chicken nuggets, and fried potatoes are the staples, so it is no surprise that people continue eating meals such as this throughout adulthood. Human beings are creatures of habit, and the habit of fried foods and melted cheese is hard to break. No wonder office lunches tend to be generally unhealthy. While offices tend to forgo McNuggets and grilled cheese for lunch, it wouldn't be hard to find office lunches featuring pizza, potato chips, or cookies.

The only way to successfully navigate office lunches is to have a plan. Plan to pack a lunch, plan to go to a healthy restaurant, or insist on salad being brought in. Employers are wising up to the fact that healthy employees take fewer sick days and have cheaper insurance policies, so they should be happy to oblige. If all else fails and there is nothing healthy to eat, you don't have to eat anything at all. Skipping lunch doesn't make you anorexic or crazy: grab a piece of fruit, keep working, and get out of work an hour earlier. Alternatively, use lunch as a time to hit the gym or go for a walk. You could eat later.

DINNER:

Dinner is the biggest opportunity to eat healthy. You are already at home and have all evening to enjoy your meal. There is less social pressure to eat certain ways because the evening is your time. Most people consume the majority of their calories for the day during this meal, and it is the easiest meal to eat healthy.

Yet how rarely is dinner actually viewed that way?

Most of the time, when you come home from work, you are hungry and tired, and the last thing you want to do is to start cooking a meal. So you end up seated in front of the TV, scrolling through Grubhub on your phone.

Again, it is always helpful to have a plan. If you prepare dinner in advance, you'll be able to eat earlier and not have to make tough decisions late in the day. Make dinner plans with friends or family around a healthy cuisine. Make a pot of chili at the beginning of the week, and have it for dinner every other night that week. Slow cookers are also great ways to have dinner waiting for you when you get home. Throw some meat and veggies in there before work, and blammo, dinner.

Alternatively, if you are the type to just go home, open the fridge, and try to figure out what to eat, here is the new strategy.

STEP 1: Open the fridge
STEP 2: Grab the first healthy thing you see
STEP 3: Eat it
STEP 4: Drink some water and figure out dinner

The purpose of this action plan is to avoid procrastination and indecision. People will find any excuse to snack. Instead, just start eating more healthy food. Keep baby carrots in your fridge along with, cottage cheese, yogurt, berries, and any variety of snack-able produce.

If all else fails, it is totally cool to snack your way through dinner. For example, you could have baby carrots and hummus for an appetizer, cottage cheese and peaches for the main course, and an apple and peanut butter for dessert. It may not be as sexy as steak, potatoes, and vegetables, but there is no preparation or cooking involved.

Instant healthy gratification.

From now on, look at your meals differently. Breakfast is still the most important, but you can eat it whenever; lunch is a glorified snack that should be planned for; and dinner is for enjoyment. Start thinking about your meals this way today, and you'll find healthy eating a whole lot easier.

CHAPTER 9
Obesity Is not a Disease

IN MODERN-DAY AMERICA, where participation trophies and politically correct language are prevalent, sometimes it's hard to talk straight with people.

You are forced to walk on eggshells when talking about any subject matter related to weight or dieting, as you don't want to create an unhealthy relationship with food or shame anyone's body type.

First, it is important to have a healthy relationship with what you eat. You must understand that, no matter how you feel about it, there is only one relationship you can possibly have with food:

If you eat too much, you gain weight, feel bloated, and suffer from joint pains.

If you eat a slight calorie deficit, you'll lose weight.

If you eat an appropriate amount of nutrient-dense food for your age, weight, and activity level, you feel healthy and have no discernible health issues caused by your diet.

That's it. Every other aspect of your relationship with food is a product of your habits, upbringing, and how you think about food.

Your body composition is something that is measurable and changeable. If you track your calorie consumption over time, you can deduce what you must consume to maintain, lose, or gain weight. You can also influence body composition by tweaking the ratio of macronutrients that you eat. Increasing muscle mass and working out allows you to increase your overall intake without gaining additional weight. It is all measurable, and results are guaranteed.

If we are going to talk about improving your body composition, the second thing we must address is body image. There is nothing healthy about feeling bad about your current body or making someone else feel bad about their body. For some people, one hundred pounds is a healthy weight; others feel good at around two hundred. As humans, we're all basically just like different types of monkeys, and our different sizes and features are simply products of our biology.

It isn't nice to call other people fat, so don't do it to yourself. If you are overweight, positive self-talk is key. Remind yourself that you are on a journey and you are doing better than the day before.

It is hard to talk to someone about weight loss; there is almost no polite way to tell someone they need to lose weight. On top of that, telling an overweight person that they're just "big-boned" isn't productive. The best strategy is to preach the benefits of a healthy lifestyle instead of the negative side of obesity. Talk about how much better they'll feel, sleep, and copulate. But challenges still abound.

Weight loss needs to be viewed as something you can control. The American Medical Association might label obesity as a disease, but that certainly isn't a healthy viewpoint for someone to have.

Unfortunately, in the politically correct America of today, obesity *is* considered a disease. To be sure, there are thyroid problems and prescription drugs that can strongly influence your weight, but in all likelihood, these rare conditions don't affect you. Obesity could be a disease in a social context—it certainly qualifies as an epidemic—but medically speaking, it does not fit the bill. Becoming overweight as a result of an unhealthy diet and lifestyle is not a disorder. Your body is reacting to stimuli (or lack thereof) exactly as it's supposed to. If you bought a plant and didn't water it and then the plant died, you wouldn't say, "There was nothing I could do; it had Lack-of-Water Disease." The same goes for people and lack of exercise and nutrients.

In addition, labeling obesity a disease may cause an individual to view their health as out of their control. It takes responsibility away from the overweight person and puts it on their doctor. The American Medical Association's decision to label obesity a disease was based on the idea that doing so would force physicians to take this epidemic more seriously. The only problem is that now one-third of the country is technically "diseased," which is a bit insulting to people with serious diseases, like the 584,000 who die of cancer each year, or the families of the 93,000 people suffering from Alzheimer's disease.

Regardless of how you categorize it, obesity is a huge problem. And while the advice that you should love your body unconditionally is a nice idea, I guarantee you won't love the litany of health problems that go along with obesity. All love is conditional—you wouldn't love your partner as much if they were cheating on you and stealing your money to bet on dog fighting every night.

Love is actually an effective weight-loss strategy, as long as you make sure to love the things that move you forward, not those that hold you back. Love working on your health, love the improvement from yesterday, and love the confidence you build.

Mental Strategies

1. You are responsible for everything that happens in your life.

You are the hero in your journey, and everything that happens to you is a result of your actions. *You are not a victim.* So don't act like one.

You cannot pawn your health off on others, claiming that you are unhealthy because of external influences in your life. Your job is "too stressful," you are "surrounded by temptation," or "it just isn't our culture" are excuses you've been telling yourself to justify your behavior.

Obesity is not a disease, because your actions dictate whether or not you suffer from it. Becoming obese is not something that happens overnight; it is a product of bad habits repeated. Nobody has ever gotten fat from eating one pizza. And no one has ever gotten skinny from one workout. Consistency is key to a health journey, and you are responsible for keeping it up. It's all on you.

It is true that some people are going to have to work much harder to get results than others, but that's not always a bad thing. The genetically gifted tend to fall victim to a vicious cycle of losing weight, followed by complete disregard for their health, which inevitably results in injury. It's the type of person who believes that at age forty they can go out and run a marathon with little or no preparation because "they've done it before."

Your body type was given to you by the luck of the draw, and, luckily, body type is more a result of consistent action than anything else. Are you naturally skinny? It might take a little longer to gain muscle. Would you consider yourself heavy set or thick (not just overweight)? It's likely you are going to respond best to weightlifting and a lower-carb diet. Are you naturally muscular? Lucky you; everything will be easier. As you age, your body type will change, and, if you don't focus on your health, you may not like the changes that occur.

2. Love your body and be patient; everything takes time. You won't succeed overnight.

Everything starts with your perception and your expectations of yourself. To have a healthy view of your health journey, you've got to love yourself and be patient. Be grateful; you've got it pretty good. And you are already making progress on your health journey by reading this book.

If Tony Robbins is right and "progress equals happiness," every little step in the right direction should feel like hugging puppies while riding a unicorn.

If it doesn't, you'll have to just be patient like the rest of us. Forgoing a cheeseburger for a salad isn't necessarily fun and won't have a major impact on your health if you do it only one time. You'll have to forgo that cheeseburger about twenty times before you notice any changes in body composition. The same is true for gaining muscle—you won't look shredded after one workout; it takes a year to gain ten pounds of muscle.

That's what makes patience and persistence the most effective tools in getting stronger and leaner. Real change takes time, and it cannot be rushed.

3. Nobody cares about how you look

Everyone is far too self-centered to care about how you look. A lot of people feel self-conscious when going to the gym or the beach because they feel like everyone is looking at them. They aren't. People are far too busy looking in the mirror to even think twice about someone else. In fact, in the gym, people's concerns are generally as follows: first, by far, themselves; second, unquestionably, their phone; and third, reluctantly, their surroundings. If you are taking steps to improve yourself, everyone there will either help you succeed or totally ignore your existence.

If you still don't feel confident in the gym, hire a personal trainer. They will teach you how to properly move your body. Good trainers are a great investment, not only because they are experts in how to move, but because they also hold you accountable. You aren't going to miss a workout if the workout costs $100. If that seems steep, well, that's because it is. However, there are many other, lower-budget options if you still would like a personal trainer. Do a half-hour session once a week with a friend. That should run you less than $30 per person. Take a group class like Zumba;

nobody looks cool doing Zumba, but it is pretty fun hitting stuff with drumsticks.

No matter what you do, you won't look sillier than the guy who films workout videos in the gym for a book. If you don't believe me, check out the workout library at *www.doitatyourdesk.com*.

4. Spend time with empowering people, and distance yourself from draining ones

You are the lowest common denominator of the people you spend the most time with.

It makes sense; people tend to adopt the habits of their closest friends. If all your friends eat pizza and ice cream on Friday nights, there is a good chance you do, too. If all your friends like playing sports, there is a good chance you also like sports. Our friends are people we can do fun activities with or spend time with enjoyably.

Making big lifestyle changes is hard, because you need to change your habits. Your habits might be activities you do with a group, like happy-hour drinks or ice-cream socials, and while those things are great in moderation, they won't help you on your health journey. You are currently in the process of devising a master plan for your health-and-wellness journey. It will be incredibly beneficial if you have some supportive friends to help you along the way. Even criminals need accomplices. Surround yourself with supportive, like-minded individuals.

Thanks to modern technology, this has never been easier. Type a healthy activity you'd like to try into the Internet machine, and schedule a time to do it. Seriously, *put it in your schedule* so you actually do it. Show up fifteen minutes early, and schmooze the regulars. If you enjoy yourself and the people, return to the same place at the same time next week. Repeat. You'll have a new crew in no time; healthy activities generally have a welcoming community filled with like-minded individuals, especially at smaller gyms.

If you are looking for a unique community, find activities that interest you online at places like meetup.com or Facebook groups. If there is an activity that interests you, chances are there is already a community built around said activity in your area. Depending on the season, there are also intramural sports. Intramural sports are great because you are held accountable to your teammates and your wallet. Intramural sports aren't cheap, and they generally have limits on the size of the team, so once you sign up, you are committed socially and financially.

Not everyone wants to go out and make new friends for their health journey, because it seems like a daunting task. However, making new friends with similar interests is actually easier than convincing your current friends to change their ways.

Replace your old habits with better ones. Instead of Friday-night beers, how about Friday-night vodka and water? Instead of ice cream, how about froyo? If your friend is unwilling to compromise in this regard, you may need to see this person less. It's a bad sign if you are trying to better yourself and your "friend" refuses to be accommodating. Not all people are supportive. You know the kind of people who complain all the time and drain the energy from a room? People who try to tempt you into drinking when you say you are driving or those rooting for your failure? You don't need to be around those types of people. You need the kind of people who leave you feeling energized; when you suggest a fun activity, they are all in before you even describe the endeavor.

Your social circle is a sacred thing; guard it closely. Your social circle influences the activities you do, your political beliefs, and your health. Do not admit people lightly.

5. Don't weigh yourself every day

Scales are not for everyone. There are plenty of reasons why. Some people become obsessive, some people can't handle the number going up, and some people simply don't care about that number.

A scale can be an effective tool for monitoring progress in a weight-loss journey. I use it with a lot of clients whose goal is weight loss. However, in an effort to prevent compulsive scale usage, I recommend weighing yourself once a week under the exact same conditions. This is a much better indicator of progress than daily weigh-ins because the change is likely less circumstantial.

If you don't take that approach, the scale can lie to you. Often your weight goes up, even though you are sticking to your diet and exercise routine. What gives?

Water weight is probably the most influential factor. If you ate a lot of salty foods yesterday, it is possible that you are bloated. Your body simply retained more water than usual.

Additionally it is possible that last night you ate a bit later than usual, and you haven't given your body sufficient time to digest and excrete the waste. Poop can be surprisingly heavy.

Weigh yourself once a week, and remember that weighing less might not be the best strategy for looking better. Muscle weighs more than fat, so if you choose to use the scale as your main measurement of success, take pictures to track your progress alongside the scale. You may find you like how you look at 160 pounds more than 150 pounds.

There is nothing wrong with wanting to look better. Looking better or "more toned" is the primary reason people give for starting their health journey. "Better" is not quantifiable, however. How much weight you can lift, how much you weigh, or even the size of your biceps are more measurable goals that you can easily track.

6. Keep a journal or notes on your phone

Are you going to remember these six things a week from today?

Let's be honest—there is only a small chance that you'll remember your goals, how much you eat in a day, your workout, along with all the other responsibilities you have in life. If you want to guarantee your success, you need some tracking system.

There are apps for tracking your food intake, journals for tracking your workouts, and spreadsheets for everything in between. It is easier to make progress when you know how many calories you eat in a day, how much weight you used in every set of your workout, and how much sleep you are getting. These things are what make for a healthy individual, and while you don't need to track everything you do for the rest of your life, writing things down is a helpful tool for making changes.

CHAPTER 10

Persistence

"NOTHING IN THIS WORLD can take the place of persistence. Talent will not: nothing is more common than unsuccessful men with talent. Genius will not: unrewarded genius is almost a proverb. Education will not: the world is full of educated derelicts. Persistence and determination alone are omnipotent." Calvin Coolidge

Our ability to live healthy, pain-free lives comes down to our habits. The little actions we take every day compound over time to allow us to reach our wellness goals. We are the results of the action we continually take, and whether those actions are good or bad doesn't change that fact.

> "Nothing in this world can take the place of persistence. Talent will not: nothing is more common than unsuccessful men with talent. Genius will not: unrewarded genius is almost a proverb. Education will not: the world is full of educated derelicts. Persistence and determination alone are omnipotent."
>
> —*Calvin Coolidge*

If you want to be stronger, you need to exercise more. If you want to lose weight, you need to focus on eating better, and if you want to live a pain-free life, you need to spend less time in compromising positions. These are non-negotiable. It is hard to create habits. It takes an immense amount of discipline initially, but after a few months, it just becomes part of your life, like brushing your teeth. It isn't about how much you enjoy it—it's just part of the routine. Building multiple new habits at once is even harder; that is why you should start with small, attainable goals.

Instead of "I'm never eating sugar again," how about. "I am going to eat a vegetable at every meal"? Instead of "I'm going to go to the gym every day," how about "I am going to do thirty minutes a day of movement outside my regular activities"? And instead of "I'm going to stand all day at work," how about, "I am going to stand less and have better sitting mechanics"?

You don't have to jump from sedentary to marathon runner. In fact, again, you definitely shouldn't try that. Take small steps toward your health goals and you'll have a much better chance of actually reaching them. Add only two little goals a month or one big-ish goal; anything more than that is overload. At the start of every new year, crowds of people flock to the health-and-fitness industry as they resolve to build on last year's failure or success; however, in the summertime, the fitness industry slows down. Why is that? Do people care less about their health in the summer? What makes January 1 so magical?

Nothing—a new year makes people feel that they have a ton of leverage to change their lives, just like after a divorce or the death of a loved one. It is a big marker in our minds that allows us to note when we started. It's an external spark of inspiration. It doesn't matter when you are reading this book—use this as your external spark of inspiration. You've already purchased this book, and, if you take any advice from it, that is a huge win for me as the author. However, if you don't take any action, you will have read a lot of pages and spent a couple dollars. That is a lot of time and a little money for no results.

Pick something easy—eat a salad a day, sleep at least seven hours a night, drink more water, but please take action. All the little habits are the building blocks of health. Most people don't change all at once; it takes time and cultivating those little habits.

If you pick up one small habit a month, a year from today you'll have twelve new positive habits. By easing into them, you'll find that they aren't too hard to maintain. Just make the positive habits manageable.

Here are a few easy ones to start. The more easy ones you can manage, the better you'll fare with the hard ones:

1. Floss in the morning.

2. Get the mail every day.

3. Make your bed every morning.

4. Do the dishes after eating.

5. Move for thirty minutes a day.

6. Watch no more than two hours of TV per day.

7. Consume no alcoholic drinks during the week.

8. Consume protein in your first meal of the day.

9. Read one book a month.

10. Meditate.

11. Don't use any electronics for an hour before bed.

12. Keep a journal (admittedly, this one isn't easy).

The possibilities are endless. Come up with a few easy habits of your own, and start building your arsenal. I wish I could take the credit for this idea, but I just tweaked what Ben Franklin did when he was trying to acquire his thirteen virtues. I'm a huge B. Frank fan. He didn't become one of the most important figures in history overnight; it took him years of continued improvement. Your goal may not be to have your face on the $100 bill, but if all it takes is baby steps, there is no reason not to aspire after large goals. Success is a habit, just like flossing; the more you do it, the more it becomes second nature. That's what makes these little habits so important. They give you the feeling of control over your life, which is so important for your self-esteem.

Start today; time passes quickly, and the older you get, the faster it moves. You don't want to end up in the same place a year from today. You have all the tools you need to live a healthy life from the comfort of your home or office; it is just a matter of implementing them.

Or don't. I'm not your mother.

Strength Test for Runners

RUNNING IS AN EXERCISE that requires a base level of strength to do without a high risk of injury. If you can complete these three exercises pain free, you have the strength to go for a run.

HIGH KNEES FOR THIRTY SECONDS:

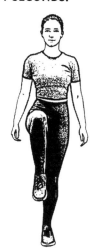

Dynamically alternate picking up your knees, barely letting your heels touch the ground.

SINGLE-LEG BOX SQUAT:

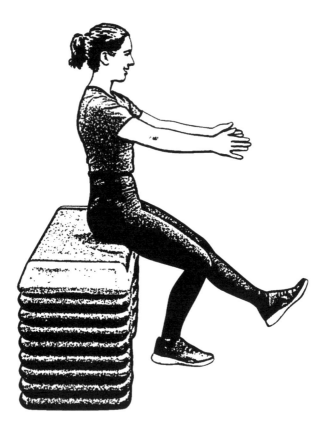

Start seated with your foot six inches away from the chair. Stand up on one leg and attempt to lower yourself back down with complete control. Try not to plop back onto the chair. Complete eight repetitions on each side.

INVISIBLE JUMP ROPE FOR ONE MINUTE:

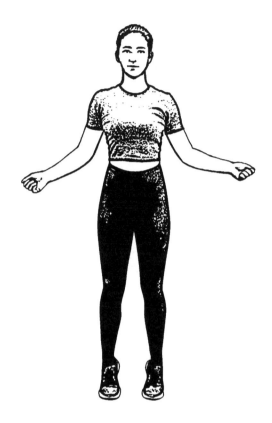

Running is essentially just one thousand little jumps, so the invisible-jump-rope test is arguably the most important test for runners. If you do not have the stamina or strength in your calves for one minute of small hops, it may not be time to pick up running.

If you can complete thirty seconds of high knees, eight single-leg box squats on each leg, and one minute of invisible jump ropes without pain, you likely have the strength necessary for running. Start with short distances on soft ground, and increase your mileage gradually.

Lower-back-pain protocol five minutes a day:

Three Rounds:

Cat/Cow x10 repetitions
Hinge Stretch x10 repetitions
Squat x10 repetitions
Bird-Dog x8 repetitions each side
Dead Bugs x8 repetitions each side

CAT/COW—Start on your hands and knees with your hands under your shoulders and knees under your hips. Look up toward the ceiling, and let your belly fall toward the floor. Move slowly and only within a pain-free range of motion.

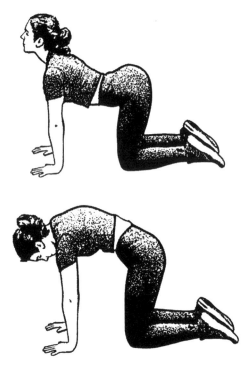

Slowly transition from the cow to the cat position by totally relaxing your neck and letting your head fall between your shoulders, simultaneously trying to bring your shoulder blades toward the ceiling. Transition to and from these positions ten times for a single set.

HINGE STRETCH—With your back flat and knees soft, try to push your butt straight back until your torso is almost parallel with the ground. Stand up, and do ten repetitions.

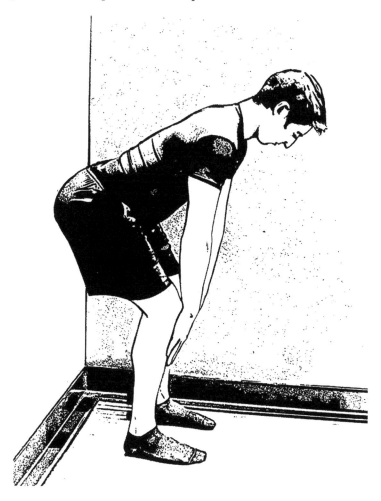

SQUAT—The squat is a strength exercise but also a great way to loosen up your lower back! Standing with your feet shoulder-width apart, try to sit as deep as you feel comfortable. Keep your feet flat on the ground and your back straight, and return to the standing position. Do ten repetitions.

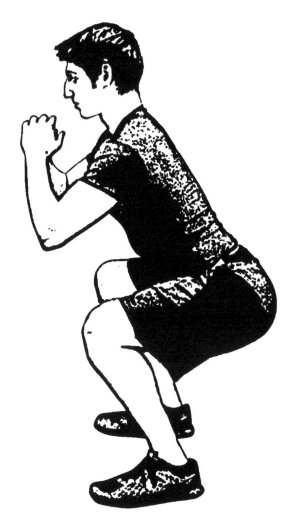

BIRD-DOGS—The bird-dog is the quintessential back exercise. It is based around maintaining a neutral spine and squared shoulders and hips while simultaneously kicking back a leg and pressing out the opposite arm. This exercise reinforces solid hip and shoulder mechanics, builds core strength, and is the complete package in back-pain prevention.

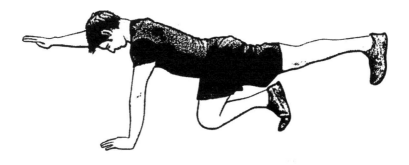

Starting from the quadruped position, hands under shoulders and knees under hips on all fours, extend the opposite arm and leg fully before returning to the starting position. Do eight repetitions on each side.

DEAD BUGS—The dead bug is an ab exercise designed to help build strength to protect your lower back. They are essentially bird-dogs on your back. Extend the opposite arm and leg fully while bracing your abs, pause, and return to the starting position. Do eight repetitions on each side.

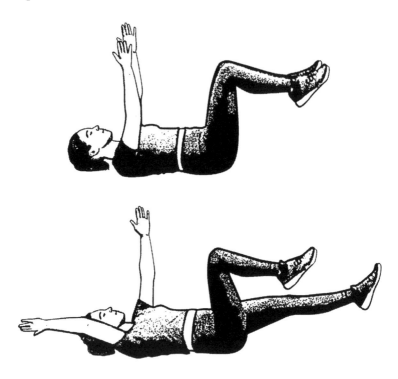

If this is too strenuous when starting out, try lifting your leg up instead of out and build up to full extension.

Upper-back-pain protocol five minutes a day:

Two rounds of:

Chest Stretch—20 seconds each side
Pocket Stretch—20 seconds each side
Trap Stretch—20 seconds each side
Foam Roll Upper Back—30 seconds

CHEST STRETCH—It may seem odd to start a workout for upper back pain with a chest stretch, but tight chest muscles can be one of the major causes of bad posture and contribute to pain in your upper back and neck.

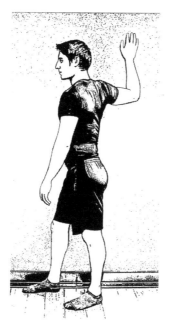

Place your arm flat against the wall and rotate your torso away from the wall.

POCKET STRETCH—Stand up straight with your chin back and maintaining your shoulder position; turn your chin toward your front pocket, and gently pull down on the crown of your head.

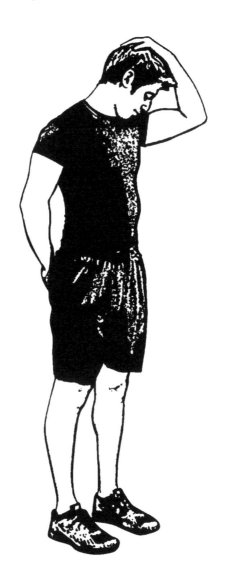

TRAP STRETCH—Stand up straight with your chin back and maintaining your shoulder position; gently pull your ear toward your shoulder.

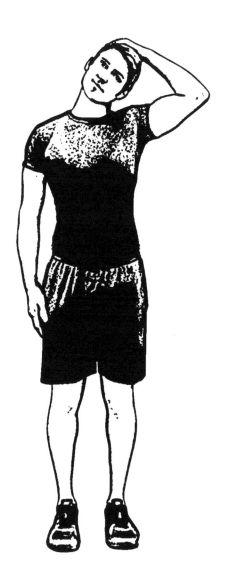

FOAM ROLL UPPER BACK—Lay on a foam roller with hands over your head, and locate tight spots on your upper back. Keep the foam roller there until the tension starts to dissipate.

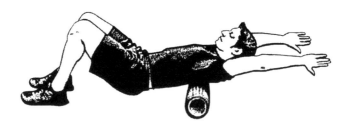

To add more pressure, lift your butt off the ground, or, if needed, place your hands behind your head to support your neck.

Super-Simple Pull-Up Progression:

Perform this routine three times per week to achieve your first pull-up in no time!

PHASE 1:

Rows—Four sets of eight repetitions (4x8)

Farmers' Walks—Four sets of forty-five seconds (4x45s)

Top of Pull-Up Hold—Four sets of max time; perform assisted with band or machine if needed (4x max)

Perform Phase 1 workouts until you can hold the top of the pull-up position for ten seconds unassisted.

PHASE 2:

Negative Pull-Ups—Four sets of three reps; lower for four seconds or as slow as possible (4x3)

Top of Pull-Up Hold—Four sets of five seconds (4x5s)

Farmers' Walks—Four sets of one minute (4x60s)

Rows—Four sets of ten repetitions (4x10)

Perform Phase 2 workouts until you can complete all of the negative pull-ups with good form at the allotted tempo.

PHASE 3:

Negative Pull-Ups—Four sets of five repetitions; lower for six seconds (4x5)

Farmers' Walks—Four sets of one minute (4x 60s)

Rows—Four sets of six repetitions; increase weight from Phase 2 (4x6)

Perform Phase 3 workouts until you can complete all of the negative pull-ups with good form at the allotted tempo.

PHASE 4:

Three-quarters range of motion pull-up—Three sets of two repetitions (3x2)

Negative Pull-Ups—Three sets of three repetitions; lower for ten seconds (3x3)

Farmers' Walks—Four sets of one minute (4x60s)

Perform Phase 4 workouts until you can complete all three-quarters range of motion pull-ups along with all of the negative pull-ups with good form at the allotted tempo.

PHASE 5:

Do a pull-up—you are ready.

ROWS—Rows can be performed in a number of different ways. There are cable rows, dumbbell rows, and TRX rows, but no matter what row you are doing, you always want good form. Set your shoulders before every rep, row only until your elbow is even with your back, and lower the weight with control.

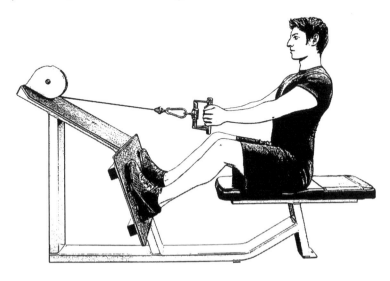

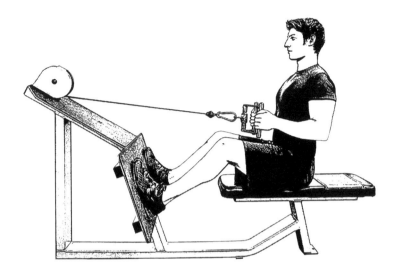

FARMERS WALKS—These mean walking with weights while keeping good posture. Keep the center of the weights in line with your ears and do not swing the weights.

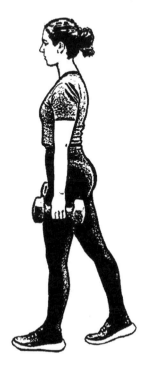
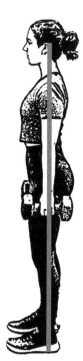

TOP OF PULL-UP HOLD—With your chest up and your shoulders down, hold the top of the pull-up position.

Imagine you are trying to put your shoulder blades in your back pocket.

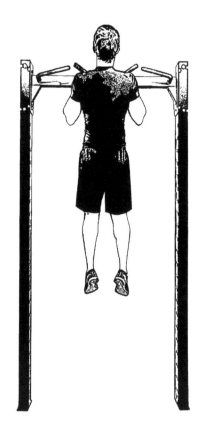

NEGATIVE PULL-UP—By jumping or using a step, start at the top of the pull-up position, and, with control, lower to hanging.

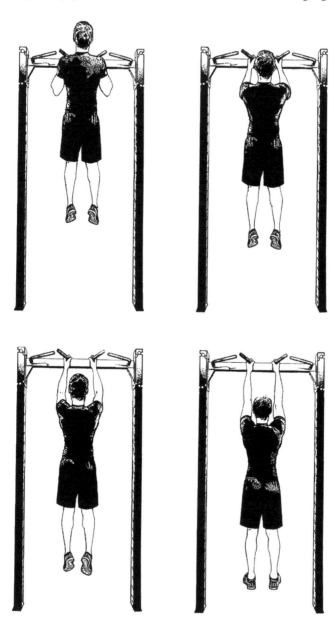

THREE-QUARTERS PULL-UP—To perform a limited range of motion pull-up, start on a box with your arms slightly bent so that you're about one fourth of the way there, and pull up the last three-fourths.

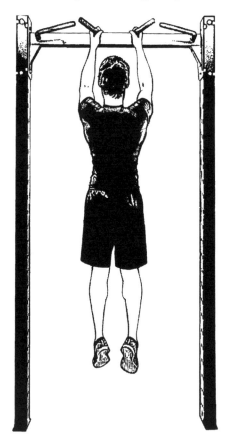

Sedentary to Strong:

The goal of this workout plan is to take you from the couch to basic strength training with a low risk of injury. Often, when starting a strength program, people will attempt to do too much too soon and get injured. But this plan is designed to keep you healthy and set you up for success in your newfound active lifestyle.

Perform each workout for a week, three to five times per week. Each workout is designed to take around fifteen minutes, so you can always fit them into your schedule with enough time to warm up beforehand.

Note:

A super set is an exercise performed back to back with the rest after both movements. For example:

1a) Deadlift 3x10
1b) Squat 3x10

This means do move A, followed by move B, rest, and then repeat that sequence three times.

As opposed to:

1. Deadlift 3x10
2. Squat 3x10

This would indicate that you should complete three sets of ten repetitions of deadlifts before moving on to squats.

PHASE 1
1a) Dead Lift Stretch 3x10
1b) Box Squat 3x10
2a) Reverse Lunge 3x8 each leg

2b) Assisted Push-Ups 3x8
3) Planks 3x30s

PHASE 2
1a) Deadlift Stretch 3x10
1b) Squats 3x10
2a) Reverse Lunge 3x10
2b) Assisted Push-Up 3x10
3a) Single-Leg High Planks 3x20 each leg
3b) Side Plank 3x15 each side

PHASE 3
1a) Bridges 3x10
1b) Squats with Hands behind Head 3x12
2a) Bulgarian Split Squats 3x6 each leg
2b) Push-Ups 3x6
3a) Planks 3x60s

PHASE 4
1a) Push-Ups 3x8
1b) Side Lunges 3x5
2a) Squats with Pause at Bottom 3x10 +2s pause
2b) Bulgarian Split Squat 3x8 each leg
3a) Dead Bugs 3x8 each side
3b) Side Plank 3x20s each side

PHASE 5
1) Single-Leg Box Squat 3x6 each leg
2) Single-Leg RDL 3x5 each leg
3a) Bulgarian Split Squats 3x10 each leg
3b) Side Lunge 3x8 each leg
4a) Dead Bugs 3x10 each side
4b) Triceps Push-Ups 3x5

PHASE 6

1a) Triceps Push-Ups 3x8
1b) Single-Leg Box Squats 3x8
2a) Single-Leg RDL 3x6 each leg
2b) Side Lunges 3x10
3a) Single-Leg High Plank 3x30s each leg
3b) Side Planks 3x25s each side

Throughout this workout, there are five types of movements: push-up, hinge, squat, lunge, and plank. Each type of movement has variations, but the principles of how the movement is performed stay the same across every variation.

PUSH-UPS (ASSISTED, TRICEPS)—Push-ups whether assisted, triceps, or otherwise, are all very similar. If at any point during the workouts you cannot do the prescribed number of repetitions, simply find a higher surface to push off of, and continue assisted.

For the push-up, start with your hands a bit wider than your shoulders, brace your abs, and imagine you are trying to keep your body in a straight line from your butt to the back of your head. Inhale, lower with control, and exhale on your way up.

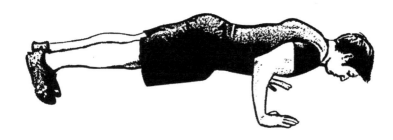

PUSH-UP—For an assisted push-up, simply perform a push-up on any elevated surface. The lower the surface, the more difficult the push-up.

ASSISTED PUSH-UP—For the Triceps Push-Up, narrow your grip to just wider than your torso and bring your elbows straight back as you lower.

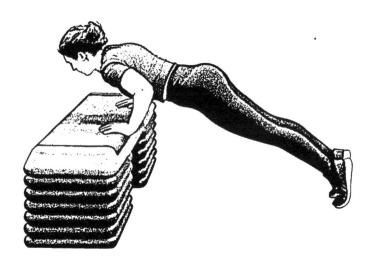

TRICEPS PUSH-UP

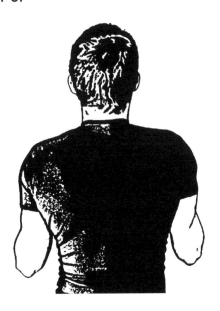

HINGE (DEAD LIFT, BRIDGE, SINGLE-LEG RDL) Hinging is a motion initiated by your hips. The goal throughout all of the hinge motions is to maintain a neutral spine while engaging your abs, hamstrings, and glutes.

DEAD-LIFT STRETCH—For the dead-lift stretch, start with your feet hip-width apart. Keep your back flat, and imagine you are trying to push your butt straight back while your shins stay as vertical as possible. Reach for the middle of your shins, and stand back up, letting your hips guide the movement.

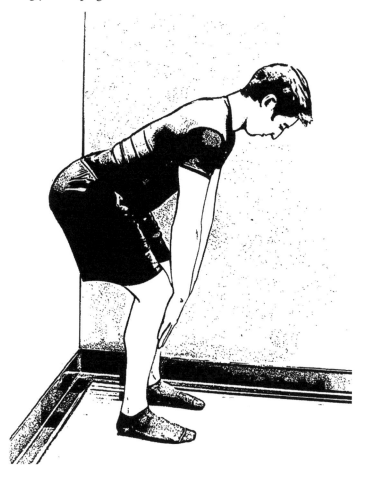

SINGLE-LEG RDL—The single-leg RDL looks difficult, but remember it's the same as the dead lift but on one leg. You are still letting your hips guide the movement while maintaining a neutral spine and bracing. For the single-leg RDL, keep your knee bent and your back foot dorsi-flexed (meaning toe pointed toward your ankle). Start standing on one leg, and finish almost parallel to the ground.

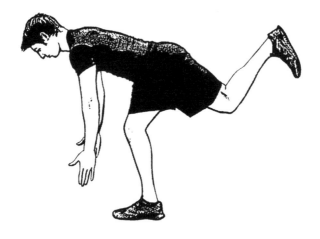

BRIDGE—Bridging is just hinging on the floor. You start lying on your back with your feet hip-width apart. Bring your hips up one vertebra at a time until you are in the position below. Brace your abs, and squeeze your glutes at the top.

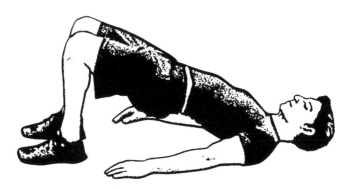

SQUAT (BOX SQUAT, SINGLE-LEG BOX SQUAT)—Start standing with your feet shoulder-width apart. Imagine you are going to try to sit in a chair. Maintain a neutral spine, drive your knees out wide, and lower until your butt touches the box or as deep as you can go with good form.

BOX SQUAT—Keep your feet as straight as possible and flat on the ground. Imagine you are trying to spread the floor apart by creating force in opposing directions as you go back up to standing.

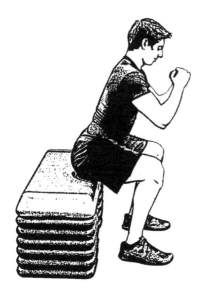
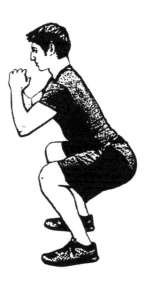

For a single-leg squat, start seated, with your foot six inches away from the chair. Stand up on one leg, and attempt to lower yourself back down with complete control. Try not to plop back onto the chair.

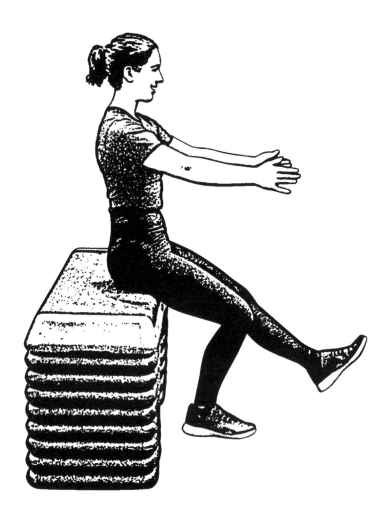

LUNGE (SIDE LUNGE, REVERSE, BULGARIAN SPLIT SQUAT)—A lunge is just like a single-leg squat. Whenever we are lunging, we are focusing on one leg. All of these exercises are almost single-leg exercises with another leg there simply for balance.

REVERSE LUNGE—To perform a reverse lunge, start with your feet hip-width apart. Imagine your feet are on railroad tracks so that they always stay in line with your hips, even when they are behind you. Take a big step back, and drop your back knee straight down. Keep your front foot flat on the ground throughout the entire movement.

To get back up, imagine driving all your weight through your front heel, and stand up.

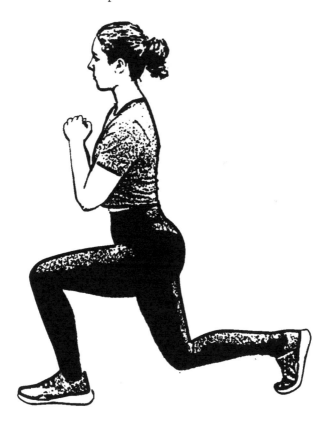

BULGARIAN SPLIT—A Bulgarian split squat is the same thing as a lunge, but there is more than one way to do it. Some people experience pain in the tops of their feet when performing this exercise, so below are two different ways to go about it. Both ways are beneficial—it is just about what feels best for you.

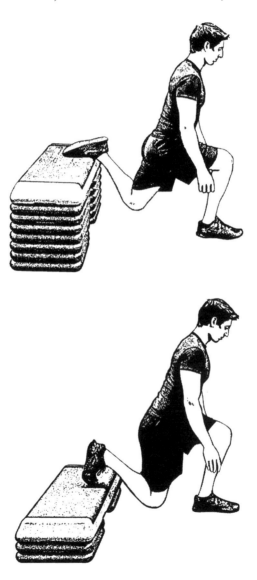

A side lunge is a lateral movement. Start standing; step out wide to one side, and totally relax your trailing leg. Bend your knee, push your butt back, and shift all your weight over the foot you just stepped with. Drive through your heel, and stand up to return to the starting position a few feet from where you started.

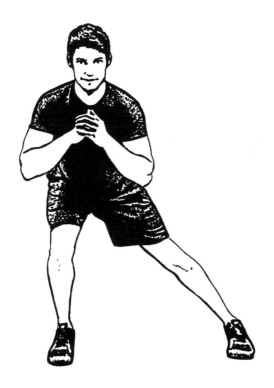

PLANK (SIDE PLANK, SINGLE LEG, DEAD BUGS)—Even though it may not look like it, there is a lot going on when performing a plank. A plank is a challenging core exercise and a great exercise for gaining the strength to prevent lower-back pain.

Start in the plank position with your feet together and your forearms parallel, like railroad tracks. Imagine you are trying to push your upper back toward the ceiling while pulling your elbows toward your toes. Pulling your elbows toward your toes forces you to brace throughout the movement.

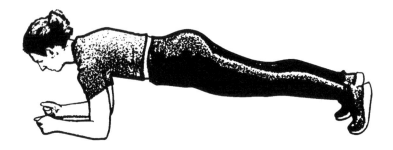

A high plank is the same thing, only on your hands. This variation is being performed with one leg in the air. Imagine you are trying to pull your hands to your toes.

SINGLE-LEG PLANK—Side planks are a beast of their own. Start on your side with your feet stacked on top of each other. Push yourself up onto your elbow and imagine you are trying to move your upper body as far away from your elbow as possible. Try to keep your body in a straight line, and don't let your hips drop to the floor.

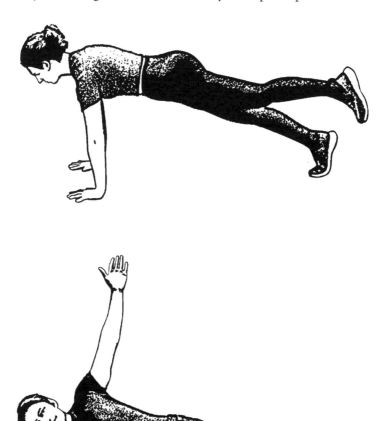

DEAD BUG—Start lying on your back with your hands and knees in the air so you look like a dead bug. Slowly extend your opposite arm and leg, pause, and return to the starting position. Next perform the same movement with the other arm and leg. Try to keep your abs braced and lower back pinned to the ground throughout the entire exercise.

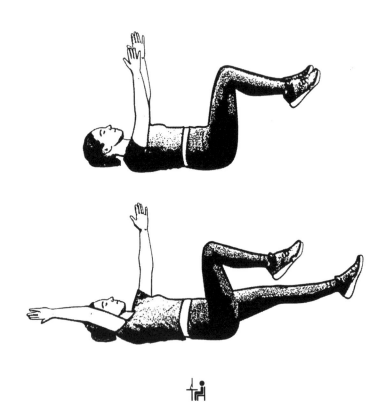

ACKNOWLEDGMENTS

AS IT TURNS OUT, it takes quite a bit of help to create a quality book, and there are many people I need to thank.

I have to start with my parents, Shelley and Ken, without whom this book would not have been possible. Not only would I not exist today to write it, but without their perpetual love and support, I doubt I'd have the confidence to share my writing. Thank you for always being in my corner from conception to publication.

This book also would not have been possible without Sharon Swanson, who tutored me in writing as a freshman in high school and helped me shape the narrative of this book. A conversation we had when I was fourteen shaped the way I viewed writing throughout my life. While working on a writing assignment that asked us to respond to one of Shakespeare's plays, I got stuck and asked, "What do I say? How am I supposed to know what to write about?" She replied, "Nobody has a freaking clue what they are talking about. Write whatever you want if you can support it." After that, I've never struggled to fill pages regardless of the subject matter.

To my wonderful, supportive girlfriend Katlyn, thank you for listening to me complain about deleting things that I've written and reminding me that quality takes time. Thank you for taking pictures, being in the pictures, and becoming a super-silly-looking illustration with me. If it weren't for you, this book might have been a long, incomprehensible mess released way before it was ready.

My sister Elana, thank you for supporting all my endeavors over the years. From elementary school, helping me raise money for a charity called "Jump Rope for Heart" in order to get the cool prize, until now, helping me sell books.

David Ellis, thank you for the vote of confidence. You are a great friend, and I am lucky to have met you during your time in Chicago. Thank you for the ongoing support.

To everyone who pre-ordered a copy of this book, thank you!

A special thank-you to those who made this book extra possible. Thank you for the contributions:

Adam Gould
Athina Koutsoumadi
Avi Schneider
Benjamin Voloshin
Beryl Rabinowitz
Colin Chisek
Cristina Anichini
Dane Hassani
David Freireich
David Ellis
Earl Hoffenberg
Edie Sue Sutker
Elana Dermer
Ethan Goldsmith
Fred Huss
Henry Chan
Howard Ankin
Ira Blumen
Jacob Ganellan

Jacob Bikshorn
James and Sharon McGowan
James Rabinowitz
Jason DiNovi
Jeff Cunix
Jennifer McGowan-Tomke
Jillian Gallagher
John Wozniak
Joshua Mintzer
Kaouther Ajroud
Karen and Allen Sutker
Katlyn Borges
Ken Dermer
Kristen Tanakatsubo
Lisa Ratajczyk
Mason Moore
Matthew Gold
Michael Arimond
Michael Miller
Michael Rosenson
Myles Kaluzna
Nancy Naleway
Rodney Camper
Ross Neihaus
Ross Kofkin
Sam Shechtman
Scott Rothschild
Scott Schreiber
Scott Engstrom
Sharon Swanson
Shelley Sutker-Dermer
Thomas Riordan
Tucker Collins
Yaakov Calamaro

I know I've asked you for a lot throughout this book, but I need to ask you for one more thing. If you enjoyed this book, would you do me a quick favor?

Like all authors, I rely on online reviews to encourage future sales. Your opinion is invaluable. Would you take a few moments now to share your assessment of my book on Amazon, Goodreads, or any other book-review website you prefer? Your opinion will help the book marketplace become more transparent and useful to all.

Sincerely,
Jake Dermer

REFERENCES

1. John Axelsson, Michael Ingre, Torbjörn Åkerstedt, Ulf Holmbäck, Effects of Acutely Displaced Sleep on Testosterone, *The Journal of Clinical Endocrinology & Metabolism*, Volume 90, Issue 8, 1 August 2005, Pages 4530–4535, https://doi.org/10.1210/jc.2005-0520

2. Dhurandhar EJ, Dawson J, Alcorn A, et al. The effectiveness of breakfast recommendations on weight loss: a randomized controlled trial. *Am J Clin Nutr.* 2014;100(2):507–513. doi:10.3945/ajcn.114.089573

3. Wendy AM Blom, Anne Lluch, Annette Stafleu, Sophie Vinoy, Jens J Holst, Gertjan Schaafsma, Henk FJ Hendriks, Effect of a high-protein breakfast on the postprandial ghrelin response, *The American Journal of Clinical Nutrition*, Volume 83, Issue 2, February 2006, Pages 211–220, https://doi.org/10.1093/ajcn/83.2.211

4. Nora Klöting, Mathias Fasshauer, Arne Dietrich, Peter Kovacs, Michael R. Schön, Matthias Kern, Michael Stumvoll, and Matthias Blüher, Insulin-sensitive obesity, *American Journal of Physiology-Endocrinology and Metabolism*, 2010 299:3, E506-E515

5. Buemann, B., Toubro, S., & Astrup, A. (2002). The effect of wine or beer versus a carbonated soft drink, served at a meal, on ad libitum energy intake. *International Journal of Obesity and Related Metabolic Disorders*, 26, 1367-1372.

6. Rixe, Jeffrey A., Gallo, Robert A., Silvis, Matthew L., 2012, Current Sports Medicine Reports, The Barefoot Debate: Can Minimalist Shoes Reduce Running-Related Injuries? https:// journals.lww.com/acsm-csmr/Fulltext/2012/05000/The_ Barefoot_Debate___Can_Minimalist_Shoes_Reduce.13.aspx

7. Torbjörn Åkerstedt, Göran Kecklund, John Axelsson, Impaired sleep after bedtime stress and worries, *Biological Psychology*, Volume 76, Issue 3,2007, pp. 170-173

8. Blumenthal JA, Sherwood A, Babyak MA, et al. Effects of Exercise and Stress Management Training on Markers of Cardiovascular Risk in Patients With Ischemic Heart Disease: A Randomized Controlled Trial. *JAMA*. 2005;293(13):1626–1634. doi:10.1001/jama.293.13.1626

9. Laukkanen T, Khan H, Zaccardi F, Laukkanen JA. Association Between Sauna Bathing and Fatal Cardiovascular and All-Cause Mortality Events. *JAMA Intern Med*. 2015;175(4):542–548. doi:10.1001/jamainternmed.2014.8187

10. Stoner L, Cornwall J. Did the American Medical Association make the correct decision classifying obesity as a disease?. *Australas Med J*. 2014;7(11):462–464. Published 2014 Nov 30. doi:10.4066/AMJ.2014.2281

ABOUT THE AUTHOR

JAKE DERMER IS THE FOUNDER of Do It At Your Desk, a company dedicated to helping office workers live healthier, more-active,

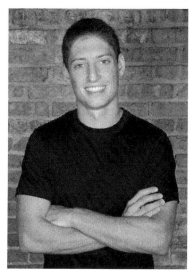

and pain-free lives. He is also a published fitness writer with a decade of experience in the personal training industry. Jake's program is the result of years of dedicated effort on helping to dispel the myths around diet and exercise. His engaging seminars and coaching motivate and inspire professionals with desk jobs to make decisions that lead to improved vitality, increased energy, and an overall sense of well-being.

Are you interested in having Jake present at your workplace? Please visit *www.DoitatyourDesk.com*

52828977R00096

Made in the USA
Lexington, KY
21 September 2019